Oriental
Breathing Therapy

Takashi Nakamura

Japan Publications, Inc.

© 1981 by Takashi Nakamura

Published by JAPAN PUBLICATIONS, INC., Tokyo and New York

Distributors:
UNITED STATES: *Kodansha International/USA, Ltd., through Harper & Row, Publishers, Inc., 10 East 53rd Street, New York, New York 10022.* SOUTH AMERICA: *Harper & Row, Publishers, Inc., International Department.* CANADA: *Fitzhenry & Whiteside Ltd., 195 Allstate Parkway, Markham, Ontario, L3R 4T8.* MEXICO AND CENTRAL AMERICA: *HARLA S. A. de C. V., Apartado 30–546, Mexico 4, D. F.* BRITISH ISLES: *International Book Distributors Ltd., 66 Wood Lane End, Hemel Hempstead, Herts HP2 4RG.* EUROPEAN CONTINENT: *Fleetbooks-Feffer and Simons (Nederland) 61 Strijkviertel, 3454 PK de Meern, The Netherlands.* AUSTRALIA AND NEW ZEALAND: *Bookwise International, 1 Jeanes Street, Beverley, South Australia 5007.* THE FAR EAST AND JAPAN: *Japan Publications Trading Co., Ltd., 1–2–1, Sarugaku-cho, Chiyoda-ku, Tokyo 101.*

First edition: September 1981
Third printing: December 1986

LCCC No. 79–91515
ISBN 0–87040–478–4

Printed in U.S.A.

Preface

Diseases can be cured by breathing. Is this really true? If such were the case, then no one in the world should be ill. This is an unconvincing statement and it is doubtful that anyone would believe it. However, before anyone makes up their mind, they should read the following.

Dr. Arthur Janov of the United States found from the blood chilling screams of neurotic patients a common anguish entrenched in their sick minds and to release this anguish, he proposed a method of treatment for neuroses involving breathing (*The Primal Scream, Primal Therapy: The Cure for Neurosis*, 1970).

Dr. D'Aiginger in Austria performs "compensated training" (Le training compensé) based mainly on breathing and has achieved major results in neurotic patients. Dr. J. H. Shultz, also an Austrian, uses breathing as one of the techniques included in "autogenic training" (Le training autogéne).

The Oriental breathing therapy introduced in this book has been performed secretly for several thousand years as one of the techniques to achieve perennial youth and immortality, an art of hermits or a method to achieve enlightenment in Buddhism, especially the Zen sect. Recently, this breathing therapy has been analyzed scientifically by various researchers including me and a system which is acceptable to modern society have been devised after many clinical trials.

The mechanism of the Oriental breathing therapy involves a conscious straining and relaxing of the muscles and nerves and also the mind through breathing. In this way, the body and mind are strengthened, resistance against disease is developed and if the person should become ill, an energy of the "spirit" is sustained to overcome the disease. The aim of this therapy is to promote a healthy body and a stable mind and bring about a complete transformation of the person both physically and mentally.

This breathing therapy is not intended to be used only as means of treating disease on a large scale, but should rather be performed freely to maintain health, prevent disease and assure a sound mind. If a person takes steps to achieve a correct posture and correct breathing, his life will greatly improve. All that is required is perseverance.

Takashi Nakamura

Contents

Preface

1. Scientific Bases of Breathing Therapy

Psychiatric Influences of Breathing on the Human Body   *11*
    The relationship between respiration and emotion   13
    The relationship between changes in mental conditions and term of expiration
        and inspiration   15
    How hyperventilation gives influence to psychology   16
Relation of Respiration Pattern to Newborn Survival   *18*
Changes in Respiration by Age   *21*
Physical Effects of Scientific Breathing Therapy   *24*
    The marked influence of breathing exercise on digestive organs   28
    Remarkable effects of breathing exercise on circulatory system   29
    Influence of breathing exercise on the nervous system   29
    Relation between respiration and capillary activity   30

2. Preparation for Breathing Therapy

Points and Purposes of Breathing Therapy   *33*
    Intentional natural breathing   33
    The number and amount of breaths   33
    Strength of breath   34
    Breathing and blood circulation   35
Principles of the Breathing Therapy   *35*
Side Effects Due to Improper Breathing Exercise and Advice against Them   *37*
Basic Postures for the Breathing Therapy   *39*
    Erect position   39
    Sitting position   47
    Lateral position   52
Seven Steps of Preparatory Exercise for the Breathing Therapy   *54*
Tension and Relaxation Exercise   *59*
Concentration of Mind   *61*
Focussing on Tanden   *62*

3. Practice of Breathing Methods

The Breathing Method That Has Been Handed Down Generation to Generation
  in the Orient   65
    "Ki" example A of the ascetic hermits   66
    "Ki" example B of the ascetic hermits   67
    "Ki" example C of the ascetic hermits   68
    "Ki" example D of the ascetic hermits   70
Outline of the Breathing Therapy   71
    The significance of deep breathing   71
    Breathing from the nose   73
    Importance of extended exhaling   74
    Relationship between breathing and the abdominal pressure   75
Nine Basic Methods for Breathing Exercise   78
    Type 1.   Rhythmical breathing method   78
    Type 2.   Prolonged breathing method   80
    Type 3.   Seven by seven breathing method   82
    Type 4.   Treble breathing method   83
    Type 5.   Snuffle-snuffle type of breathing method   86
    Type 6.   Broken wind breathing method   89
    Type 7.   Windup breathing method   91
    Type 8.   Pit and corn breathing method   94
    Type 9.   High-tension breathing method   96
Six Steps in Authentic Oriental Breathing Therapy   99
    Step 1   (Learning the method of lengthen the respiratory cycle)   100
    *Step 2   (To draw in the abdomen during expiration and push it out
      during inspiration)*   103
    Step 3   (To master even thinner and longer respiration than in Step 2)   106
    Step 4   (Back to the pattern of natural breathing)   108
    *Step 5   (Involves a breathing exercise to maintain health and immunity
      to various illnesses)*   109
    *Step 6   (Thoracic respiration no longer used, and navel used for taking
      breaths)*   109

4. Reinforcing What Has Been Achieved by the Breathing Exercises

Auxiliary Breathing Exercises   *113*
    Tapping the abdomen (effective to relax muscles and relieve fatigue)   *113*
    Yajirobei *exercise*   *115*
    *Exercise for twisting the body using waist and feet (to promote activities
      of stomach and intestines)*   *116*
    Exercise for shaking the body   *117*
    Rowing boat exercise   *118*
    Exercise for carrying a ball   *120*

Exercise for pulling legs up out of marsh   *122*
Exercise in Sumo *crouching posture*   *123*
Physical exercise with bar   *125*
Rhythmical exercise   *127*
Five Stances Designed to Promote the Effectiveness of Breathing Exercises   *129*
Tiger stance   *129*
Deer stance   *131*
Bear stance   *132*
Monkey stance   *132*
Bird stance   *132*
Massage and Shiatsu   *135*
Massage and shiatsu treatment   *140*
Mental Attitude for Undertaking Breathing Exercise   *147*
Performance of breathing exercise must be organized   *149*

Conclusion

Idea of new method of respiration   *151*
A trial for new breathing therapy   *152*

Index

1. Scientific Bases of Breathing Therapy

Psychiatric Influences of Breathing on the Human Body

Since the days of ancient Greece, circa 500 B.C., men have demonstrated a keen interest in the unknown. They have striven to investigate and have succeeded in untangling many mysteries since the dawn of history and their findings have contributed greatly to the evolution of science and technology.

Among the many things that have aroused human curiosity—nature, the universe, celestial spheres, etc.—the human body has proven to be of the most interest. Like little children, fascinated by their bodies, men have tried pulling, twisting and pinching ears and other extremities and occasionally, have been surprised by the pain which they have experienced. Men have been intrigued by the tactile sensations which result from bringing hands and fingers into contact with other parts of the body such as the mouth, the nose, the ears and the eyes, etc. Such gestures remain common to infant children throughout the world.

A large number of scientists and medical experts have been engaged continuously, for a long period of time, in basic research to solve the mysteries of the human body and its structure. Especially perplexing have been the questions of why the men are born and why they sicken and die.

Many questions raised by medical experts in their studies already have been solved. Several centuries of laborious studies have revealed an especially large amount of information about the functioning of the human body, a mysterious structure once regarded by medical experts as a black box. The causes of many once-fatal diseases have been identified and they have been forever eliminated as a threat to mankind. Researchers also have made considerable progress in their studies of human life. Intensive studies on genetic inheritance, a subject central to all theories relating to the origin of life have produced marvelous results. In Britain, medical experts have succeeded in causing the birth of a baby conceived in a test tube. It truly can be said that, in deciphering the secret genetic code, this latest round of medical research has uncovered some of the deepest mysteries surrounding human life and has shed light on the domain of the Creator himself.

While research on life itself and on the world of the material has continued in the foregoing pattern, research on the human spirit and human emotions also has progressed. Unsolved mysteries remain, however, with respect to why humans experience delight or grief and trouble, with respect to why emotional stress often becomes the cause of illness and with respect to whether there is any way to recuperate from emotional illness. Although studies to the human spirit and human emotions have been intensive, the importance of the basic relationship between breathing and physical and mental function until recently has been largely ignored. Because breathing was something common to everyone, respiratory functions were, for a long period, disregarded as appropriate subjects for scientific inquiry. One actually might say that it was breathing's importance—the universally recognized fact that, if the respiratory organs cease to function, death will follow immediately—which discouraged men from studying it. Lao Tze, an ancient Chinese sage, once said: "Men can not see the square shape as it is, if it is too big for them." It might be correct to say that breathing is "a square too big for men to see."

Dr. Wilhelm Wundt (1832–1920) attempted, during the late nineteenth and early twentieth Centuries, to explore the mysterious relationship between breathing and mental activities. Dr. Wundt and his colleagues at Leipzig University in Germany concentrated their efforts on the respiratory changes which are caused by changes in mental state. Among their works are: P. Mentz, *Die Wirkung Akustischer Sinnesreize auf und Atmung in W. Wundt*, Philosophische Studien, 1895, 11, 61, P. Zoneff and E. Maumann, *Über Bogleitersheinungen Psychischer Vorgänge in Atem und Puls in W. Wundt*, Philosophische Studien, 1903, 15, 1. and F. Rehwodt, *Über Respiratorische Affektsymptome in W. Wundt*, Psychologische Studien, 1912, 7, 141.

After the Vietnam War, U.S. medical experts engaged in extensive studies on respiration. It was found that if men breathed deeply, a substance called "endorphin" appeared in their blood streams. It was discovered that endorphin affects the cerebral cortex and helps men to forget and to eliminate fears and terror from their memory, and that it also works consistently and effectively to control and regulate the function of various human organs. As a result, endorphin was found to be effective in maintaining both mental and physical comfort. Further research has revealed that heroin stimulates the production of endorphin. However, heroin is a dangerous toxic drug and, as is well known, its habitual use is best avoided.

In the U.S., exercises which help to regulate breathing functions, such as Buddhist contemplation, practiced by those of the Zen sect, Yoga exercise and Chinese martial arts, are being viewed with renewed interest. In the Oriental countries, however, such as Japan, India and China, time-honored therapeutic methods designed to regulate and control breathing have been practiced for several thousand years. For example, in India, Yoga instructs that the purpose of the exercise of inhaling air is to absorb living power called *Prana*. "Prana" means the vitality which abounds throughout the universe. In China, also, it was believed that the purpose of inhaling air into the human body was to absorb powerful energy capable of sustaining life. In Japan's earliest written history the legendary *Nihon*

Shoki, there is a line that "the pantheon of deities" are given birth "amid a scene of a fog setting in and the wind howling just as if the air heaved a great sigh." Breathing was thus held to be of the utmost important and was taken to be the fundament of mankind. In Europe as well, expiration signified death and inspiration signified spiritual sensation and the stirring of the soul. It might well be said that this confirms that people of Europe, who gave birth to the English language, possess the same sense as Oriental peoples of the significance of breathing.

Recently, in many of the more industrially advanced nations, respiration has been the subject of extensive research efforts. A large number of findings have been published and circulated among those in the medical profession. These findings have established the fact that respiration plays a key role in the maintenance of health.

Before proceeding to the main issue of this discussion, breathing therapy, let us study further the complicated mechanism of respiration in order that we may better appreciate the effect of this breathing therapy.

The relationship between respiration and emotion

We human beings breathe continuously for as long as we live; ordinarily, 18 times in a minute, 1,080 times in an hour and 25, 920 times in a day. Breathing is normally an unconscious act, undertaken only in response to the body's physiological need to exchange gas. Various studies on respiration have revealed, however, that there is close relationship between regular, unconscious breathing and a person's emotional state.

It has been established that there is a relationship between changes in actual state of mind and changes in the rate of respiration. One experiment was conducted using six women. One was an actress trained in the ability to make her expressions match her feelings. The five remaining women were trained to make their expressions identical with that of their actress colleague who was responsible for taking the initiative in changing their expressions. In this experiment, it was found that even though the five women were asked only to mimic their leader's expression, their respiration rates decreased and tidal volume increased when they were asked to affect pleasant expressions as compared with situations in which they were requested to make unpleasant expressions. The ratio of the inspiration to expiration in each respiration, the inspiration/expiration ratio (I/E), was larger when pleasant expressions were made than when unpleasant feelings were expressed. In each instance, pleasant and unpleasant, the time required for the inspiration of each breath was found to be about the same but the time required for expiration was found to vary widely depending on whether the expression being made was pleasant or unpleasant. This indicates that expiration bears a closer relationship to changes in emotion than does inspiration. The human body appears to become more comfortable when expressing a pleasant feeling than when expressing an unpleasant feeling.

In another experiment, it was demonstrated that breathing is profoundly affected by frustration. In this case, the subject was bound to a chair after having had cowhage, a substance which causes intense itching, spread on his back. The subject was instructed not to move at all. He immediately experienced an intense itching sensation and, his instructions notwithstanding, was all but overcome by the urge to rub his back against the back of the chair. As the itching sensation intensified the subject struggled to resist the urge to scratch, his breathing became more rapid, his inspiration to expiration ratio increased erratically and he began to pant. However, once the subject resigned himself to the fact that relief would not be forthcoming from anyone else, the itching sensation began to subside, his respiration rate began to decrease, the depth of his expiration, relative to that of his inspiration, began to increase gradually and his normal breathing pattern gradually was restored.

The following observations, made during an X-ray examination, indicate that there is a correlation between diaphragm movement and changes in emotional state. It turned out in previous experiment that an initial bronchoscopic examination of the subject had revealed that the size of his bronchial cavity varied in response to pleasant and unpleasant stimuli. Subsequent X-ray examination confirmed that exposure to such stimuli caused marked changes in the range of the subject's diaphragm movements.

The subject in question had been visiting the hospital where the observations were made on a regular basis as an outpatient. His symptoms were invariably vague and, although he always complained of discomfort in his head, chest and abdomen, doctors familiar with his case attributed his difficulties to his economic situation. At the beginning of the X-ray examination the subject's diaphragm evidenced only limited movement, within a range of $\frac{1}{2}$ inch. Thereafter, the subject was instructed by those making the observations to imagine that he had found 10,000 yen (about $50) in cash while walking along the street in front of the hospital after having left the clinic. At the mere suggestion of such a pleasant prospect, the range of movement of the subject's diaphragm increased to 3-$\frac{1}{2}$ inchs. During the next phase of the experiment, the subject was instructed to imagine that the newly found 10,000 yen note had been blown away by strong winds and had disappeared. This unpleasant thought precipitated a reduction in the range of the subject's diaphragm movement to $\frac{1}{3}$ inch.

The foregoing observations suggested the existence of a strong correlation between perception of pleasantness and unpleasantness and the range of diaphragm movement. Obviously, during the course of X-ray examination, the subject was not instructed to employ any specific breathing methods. Nor was he told what organs were the subject of the examination. It is unlikely, therefore, that the subject was aware of the researcher's interest in his respiratory organs. For these reasons, the observations made during the examination were regarded as objective and reliable.

In order to confirm the initial observations, additional experiments were conducted on four other patients who were all in economic situations similar to that of the first subject. Three of the four subjects showed similar responses. X-ray examination revealed that their diaphragm movements reacted sharply to changes in the topics of discussion. However, identical X-ray examination of the fourth subject failed to show any similar reaction in diaphragm movement. This patient also did not show any similar reaction with other patients. In simultaneous, bronchoscopic examinations, administered to all subjects, the fourth subject's bronchial tube failed to show any of the signs of the relaxation or constriction demonstrated by those of the others. The fourth subject was later diagnosed by psychiatric experts as being schizothymic.

From these experiments, it became apparent that the pattern of diaphragm movement is highly sensitive to changes in suggested or imagined situations which are capable of evoking forceful emotional responses and that variations in diaphragm movement are directly related to the rate of respiration and to the amount of ventilation which is achieved by each breath. A wide amplitude in diaphragm movement results in deep, slow breathing while a narrow range of diaphragm movement results in a pattern of respiration which is shallow and rapid.

The relationship between changes in mental conditions and term of expiration and inspiration

In this experiment, three different types of pain impetus tests were conducted on two groups of patients who were suffering from mental diseases. A total of fifty patients were divided into group "A" consisting of eight males and seventeen females who had been diagnosed as hysteria, phobia and anxiety neuroses, and group "B," consisting of fifteen males and ten females who had been diagnosed as hypochondriasis, reaction melancholia and compulsive neuroses as well as schizophrenia. A fifteen-member control group "C," consisting of six males and nine females of post-graduate medical students, who had been diagnosed as no nervous diseases also was identified.

Three kinds of pain impetus, an intradermal injection of from 0.5 to 1.0 cubic centimeters of saline solution into the deltoid muscle, a sharp pinch on the elbow and a weak electrical shock to the fingertip, were administered to each of the subjects in each of the three groups in order to test the subjects' Minute Respiration Cycles (MRC) (number of respirations/minute). In each case, the experiment was conducted in the following sequence:

Stage I: Preparation (five minutes)—Baseline MRC measured;
Stage II: Alcohol Preparation (one minute)—Surface of skin, where pain impetus was to be applied, disinfected with alcohol; (two minute interval)—Rest;
Stage III: Pain Impetus (three minutes)—Pain impetus applied;
Stage IV: Relaxation (three minutes)—Subjects permitted to rest;
Stage V: Reminiscence (after three minutes of relaxation)—Subjects asked to recall feeling during application of pain impetus.

MRC measurements were made throughout Stages I through V. The findings of the experiments were as follows:

Stage	I	II	III	IV	V
Group A	18.95	19.93	25.03	20.25	22.08
Group B	18.63	18.18	19.38	18.98	18.88
Group C	17.55	17.13	19.83	18.70	19.18

The findings indicated that both groups A and C reacted in similar patterns, while only group B demonstrated a markedly different pattern of response to the experiment. Therefore, it might be permissible to say that this represented that those patients belonging to group B were believed to have been staying in another world from that the groups A and C people were living in throughout the experiment period.

On the other hand, those people belonging to group A showed rather sharp reaction to the test as compared with those belonging to group C. And this gave the lesson that the patients of group A were oversensitive and nervous and were person of strong emotion.

How hyperventilation gives influence to psychology

In this experiment, five young high school students, all in sound health, were tested to determine the affect of hyperventilation on human psychology. The subjects were asked to take deep breaths for two minutes, at a rate of 30 breaths per minute, and were then directed to rest for the ensuing three minutes. Following the rest period, they were asked to breathe by means of abdominal contraction for two minutes. This sequence, two minutes of deep breathing, followed by three minutes of rest, followed in turn by two minutes of abdominal breathing, was repeated until each of the subjects had performed a total of eight minutes of abdominal breathing. During the three minute rest intervals, the subjects were asked to take a seat and to undergo a Rorschach Test. Additionally, 5 cubic centimeters of arterial blood were drawn from each of the subjects some twenty minutes after the first round of deep breathing had begun. The researchers carefully examined these samples to determine the partial pressures of oxygen and carbon dioxide and to estimate blood pH (acidity). Finally, two urine samples were collected from each subject—one was taken an hour before hyperventilation test began, while the subjects were at rest, the other was taken one hour after the beginning of the test. In each case, the researchers recorded the volume of urine discharged and estimated its pH.

Analysis of the blood taken after the fourth round of the test was completed disclosed an estimated pH ranging from a low of 7.55 to a high of 7.80, with 7.66 being average. Carbon dioxide partial pressure ranged from a low of 11.4 mm/Hg to a high of 28.4 mm/Hg, with 15.6 mm/Hg being average, while oxygen partial pressure ranged from a low of 94.8 mm/Hg to a high of 120 mm/Hg, with

112.3 mmHg being average.

Urinalysis of the sample taken one hour before the hyperventilation test began disclosed an estimated urine pH ranging from a low of 6.05 to a high of 6.40, with 6.22 being average. However, the urine collected just one hour after the test had started was found to have an estimated pH ranging from a low of 6.20 to a high of 7.10, with 6.69 being average. Thus, from the analysis it appeared that the average estimated pH increased by 0.64 after the abdominal breathing test started. The total volume of urine discharged also was found to have increased by 53.4 cc from 92.6 cc to 146 cc after the test was administered. Blood pH on occasions is strongly adjusted within a range of 7.30 to 7.50. When pH exceeds 7.60 hyperventilation tetany takes place. In this study, heights of 7.8 were recorded but the average was 7.66.

Therefore, it is possible that the five students who were the subjects of this experiment were already suffering from hyperventilation tetany despite having taken deep breaths.

In the Rorschach Test, which was conducted during the three minute recess periods, Rorschach International Cards No. I, II and X were employed. During the first round of three minute recesses, Card No. I was exhibited to the subjects; Card No. II was exhibited during the second round; and Card No. X was exhibited during the third round of recess periods. Exhibition time was limited to the three minutes of the recess period and all the data was collected for comparison against data collected under ordinary conditions two weeks after the test was completed.

Test results and observation: Increased findings were observed in aggregate indexes (R), total reaction (W), abnormal partial reaction (Dd+S), inanimate locomotor responses (m), morphological responses (F), animal locomotor responses (A) and in types of the nature of responses. Human movement responses (M) decreased and the morphological level of (F) clearly deteriorated.

It was possible to find from the above results a characteristic emotional change in hyperventilation. In other words, a uniform tendency could be found in the forms of response appearing at times of anxiety and stress and a degree of a state of intelligence deterioration as well.

Furthermore, when observation is made of the effect of hyperventilation on diaphragm movement, examination by thoracic fluoroscopy when stimulating hyperventilation revealed that hyperventilation intensified and vertical diaphragm movement diminished in conformity to increase ventilation volume per minute and finally virtually disappeared. It was clear, that is to say, that there was a transfer to completely thoracic respiration. On this basis it is clear that hyperventilation gives rise to a variety of complaints and can also psychologically predestine states of anxiety and other emotional stress or that a transfer takes place to the thoracic respiration.

Examples of the relationship between indeterminate complaints and hyperventilation: In this case, the patient, a thirty-five years old, unmarried male employee of a local government agency, 175 centimeters tall and weighing 58 kilo-grams complained about his poor health, saying that his physical condition had deteriorated over the past ten years and that he felt languid and often irritable. He also admitted to having experienced a severe stiffening in his shoulders and, sometimes, numbness in his fingers and hands. This man said that he thought he was suffering from a serious illness and that his uneasiness had kept him from sleeping well at night. The man expressed his desire to go to a hot spring spa or a resort town some day for a week-long vacation. He hoped that, with this vacation and the therapeutic effect of a change of air, his health might improve. Unfortunately, because of his busy schedule, he had had no chance to take such a vacation, but was anxious to do so at the earliest possible date.

Physical examination disclosed the following: an estimated blood pH of 7.80, a partial pressure of carbon dioxide of 28.4 mm/Hg, a partial pressure of oxygen of 112.3 mm/Hg, an estimated urine pH of 7.10, a MRC of 27 respirations/minute, minute ventilation capacity of 10.26 liters and a tidal volume at 0.38 liters. The patient was found to have typical thoracic respiration, but was diagnosed as hyperventilation alkalosis since he was exhaling an excessive amount of carbon dioxide.

Further, examination of this patient also suggested possible correlations be-tween hyperventilation and gastrospasm, hyperventilation and weakness in hearing, and hyperventilation and decrease in visual power.

Relation of Respiration Pattern to Newborn Survival

According to clinical research, 60–70 percent of normaly pregnant women com-plain to their doctors that they experience some difficulty in breathing. However, these women's conditions are rarely serious enough to require special treatment such as the oxygen inhalation. On occasion, this puzzled not only patients but the obstetrics staff in attendance and confused diagnosis. It is said that this resulted in even greater anxiety in the pregnant women and in even greater breathing stress.

Heretofore, it was believed that pregnant women experienced a reduction in vital capacity, since the movement of their diaphragms was restricted by the enlargement of their uteri. However, recent clinical research has indicated that the vital capacity of women actually tends to increase during pregnancy, especially during the second trimester. Studies have revealed an increase of 15 percent during this period and an increase of 9 percent during the later stage, with the peak of vital capacity being reached between the 28th and 36th week of pregnancy.

Functional residual capacity: Considering the fact that vital capacity actually increases during pregnancy, it is now believed that labored respiration among pregnant women is caused not by a lack of oxygen, as was once believed to be the case, but rather, by the psychological pressures associated with being pregnant. There is a tendency for pregnant women to hyperventilate unconsciously. As a result, they experience anxiety which, in turn, aggravates their shortness of breath. They can become locked in a vicious cycle.

What is the reason for the remarkable increase in vital capacity during pregnancy? Perhaps the explanation lies in the mechanism of function of residual capacity. Specifically, it appears that a substantial decrease in residual capacity causes an increase in vital capacity. Extensive research carried out on pregnant women, both before and after pregnancy, revealed that their mean tidal volume, functional residual capacity, residual volume, and total lung capacity had decreased considerably, that their MRC had fallen slightly, and that in the later period of pregnancy, the women were found to have been hyperventilating unconsciously.

Women in labor characteristically exhibit a pattern of deep breathing called valsalva breath holding. It had been assumed that this type of respiration facilitated the consumption of large volumes of oxygen. It now appears, however, that women in labor consume less oxygen than had been anticipated. The volume of oxygen consumed per minute increases during periods of uterine contraction, but returns to a normal level during periods of uterine relaxation. Clinical research indicates that the volume of oxygen consumed is not much greater than that consumed while engaging in moderate physical exercise. Thus, it is perhaps permissible to conclude that labored respiration during pregnancy actually is caused by the variety of social, economic and domestic burdens that confront pregnant women and new mothers.

Newborn babies undergo drastic physical and physiological changes during the first few days after birth. The respiratory organs are among those internal organs which demonstrate the most marked change. Newborns must successfully make the transition from bronchial to pulmonary respiration. While passing through the birth canal, babies must accomplish a metamorphosis which is, in certain respects, equivalent to that which takes place when a tadpole changes into a frog.

While in womb, fetuses accomplish respiration through the placenta, which Dr. Walter Needham described, some 300 years ago, as "the lung in the womb." Immediately after birth, however, newborn babies must begin to breathe with their own lungs. In humans, the lungs are fully developed by about the 28th week of pregnancy. By that time, embryonic thoracic pressure is equivalent to that of the atmosphere. While the baby remains in the womb, the alveoli of lungs are filled with amniotic fluid which moves in rhythmic tidal flow resembling the flow of air during respiration. Since fetal lungs do not operate as gas exchangers, this motion bears no relation to respiratory function. It is clear, however, that babies exhibit basic, respiration-like movement during prenatal life.

One might wonder what becomes of the amniotic fluid contained in the fetal lungs during the birth process. A series of clinical studies has revealed the amniotic fluid contained in the lungs is expelled through the mouth and nose as the baby's head passes through the birth canal. The positive pressure within the canal reaches as high as 95 cm/H_2O as the head of the baby goes through it, but full immediately thereafter to zero or perhaps, even negative pressure. Not surprisingly, in certain cases of birth by cesarean section, the newborn baby experiences difficulties in expiration and sometimes has to eject a large volume of amniotic fluid from its lungs. A baby who has not been delivered through the birth canal has not been exposed to the same strong positive pressures as a baby born in the conventional way. Thus, it would appear that the squeezing of amniotic fluid out of the baby's thorax is one of the benefits to be derived from natural childbirth and its attendant strong positive pressure.

A newborn baby takes its first breath as a result of the negative interior pressure created in the thorax during the birth process. Immediately after birth, the thorax, which has been tightly compressed by positive pressure of up to 95 cm/H_2O within the birth canal, expands to its normal state and regains its original volume. This expansion creates a negative pressure within the thorax of from 10–70 cm/H_2O, allowing air to enter the lungs through the bronchi—the first inspiration in the new baby's life. The volume of this first inspiration is about 20–70 ml. which is far greater than the 15–25 ml. tidal volume of each respiration during the 24–48 hours immediately following birth.

The respiration of a normal, full-term baby usually stabilizes within the first 24 hours after the birth at a rate of about 40 respirations per minute (minute respiration cycle or MRC of 40), each with a tidal volume of from 12 to 20 ml. However, premature infants may require 72 hours or more before their respiration stabilizes, ordinarily, at a rate of about 60 respirations per minute (MRC of 60) with an average tidal volume of from 10 to 15 ml.

Premature infants fall into two categories depending upon the character of their respiration. One group is comprised of those infants with an initial MRC of greater than 60, but whose rate falls gradually with the passage of time. The other group consists of those infants whose MRC gradually increases by 25 to 100 percent above the initial MRC of the first one hour immediately following birth during the next 24 hours.

Clinical statistics indicate that, excluding those infants suffering from serious diseases, about two-thirds of all premature infants fall into the former category, while about one-third fall into the latter. It is believed that the increased rate of respiration among premature infants in the second group is caused by acidosis which is, in some cases, incompensable. About one-half of the infants in this group exhibit strong symptoms of cyanosis, a bluish coloration of the skin caused by a lack of oxygen in the blood. The mortality rate among them is about 25 percent during the first week after the birth.

There may be both actual and symbolic significance, in terms of the fundamental importance of the role of respiration, in these clinical findings with respect to the relationship between respiration rates and patterns and survival rates among newborn infants.

Changes in Respiration by Age

Human beings pass through many stages between their births and their deaths an average of some seventy-old years later. During the developmental stage, boys and girls follow markedly distinct courses in the development of their respective breathing patterns. For instance, during the compulsory education period, among children ranging in age from seven to fourteen, boys tend to have a more highly developed lung function than girls of equivalent age. Specifically, girls nine to eleven years of age generally tend to have a respiratory capacity which is 10 percent less than that of boys in the same age group. By the age of twelve, the differential between boys' and girls' respective respiratory capacities has widened to an average of 20 percent. This difference persists until the age of fourteen. Medical experts attribute the large differential between girls and boys, principally, to the internal secretion of sex hormones, especially, testosterone, a male sex hormone believed to play a key role in promoting muscle development and consequently, respiratory capacity among boys.

Studies also have been conducted to compare the lung functions of boys and girls of the same age but from different areas of Japan. The subjects were picked from two different districts—one group from the Tokyo and the other from the Nagano Prefecture in central Japan. The Tokyo group represented was representative of pupils from large cities; the Nagano group represented boys and girls from the country.

According to this study, among boys ranging in age from seven to eleven, elementary and secondary school pupils from the rural area showed an average respiratory capacity superior to that of those young boys raised in the urban district. But in the case of those boys age twelve and older, the situation was reversed in favor of those raised in Tokyo. Students from the urban area showed an average respiratory capacity superior to that of students from the rural area by a wide margin. Among girls, the respiratory capacities of the urban and rural groups showed similar trends within each age group.

These studies support the conclusion that the respiratory superiority of rural boys under the age of eleven is attributed to their generally superior physiques which, in turn, is attributed to the hard physical labor associated with the farm chores which young, pre-school boys, six years of age or younger, are required to perform in rural areas. The respiratory superiority of the boys from Tokyo in the twelve to fourteen age group, on the other hand, is attributed to the fact that boys in the urban area are believed to attain puberty at a far earlier age than those in the rural area.

A similar explanation is offered to account for the fact that in a similar study, conducted on two groups of youngsters, ages fifteen to seventeen, from Tokyo and Nagano Prefecture, respectively, no significant differences were found. It is believed that, in this case, all of the adolescent, high school students in both areas had reached puberty by the age in question.

The foregoing and a similar series of studies conducted on subjects who had already reached adulthood indicate that the general respiratory capacity of men improves constantly through late adolescence, until the age of between eighteen and twenty. After that period, however, capacity decreases gradually from year to year. By way of example, using the average figure for eighteen to twenty year-olds as an index of 100, vital capacity (VC) per square meter of lung surface was found to decline as follows:

> 95.9 for men 20–23 years old, 90.17 for men 32–34 years old, 86.07 for men 41–43 years old, 81.86 for men 51–53 years old, 76.36 for men 56–60 years old, 67.38 for men 61–65 years old, 60.48 for men 71–75 years old and 56.24 for men 75–80 years old.

Similarly, using the average figure for eighteen to twenty year-olds as an index of 100, men in the same age groups suffered a decrease in maximum ventilatory capacity (MVC) per square meter of lung surface as follows:

> 91.64 for those 20–23 years old, 86.39 for those 32–34 years old, 82.52 for those 41–43 years old, 73.91 for those 51–53 years old, 66.79 for those 56–60 years old, 63.67 for those 61–65 years old, 49.44 for those 71–75 years old and 41.7 for those 75–80 years old.

On the basis of these studies, it may be said that pulmonary functions reach a peak during the early part of life, between the ages of eighteen and twenty.

From the foregoing studies, it appears that the respiratory functions of men sixty years of age and older are, on average, inferior to those of children nine years of age. Symptoms of respiratory senility seem to manifest themselves in men during their late forties. In women, these signs tend to appear some ten years earlier than in men. It happens that the appearance of these signs seem to coincide with the appearance of the signs of aging in the muscle tissue of the human body. It is, therefore, most important for middle-aged people to master the techniques necessary to maintain respiratory capacity for as long as possible.

The most effective way to prevent the exacerbation of aging phenomena is for a person to learn how to maintain a regular respiration cycle and to rejuvenate himself by taking regular breathing cycles. This way of exercise is more useful to rejuvenate than outdoor exercises like jogging and track and field athletics which many people take for the purpose of wearing off surplus fat.

Average Maximum Ventilatory Capacity and Vital Capacity by Age Group
(Figures are for one square meter of body surface.)

Age	Vital Capacity (cc)	Maximum Ventilatory Capacity (1/min)
8	1,640±206	46.0±10.1
9–11	1,800±266	59.9± 8.6
12–14	2,130±273	61.8±12.2
15–17	2,570±337	78.3±17.7
18–19	2,770±687	81.2±15.4
20	2,660±475	79.0±16.3
21–22	2,574± 58	73.4± 2.0
23–25	2,519± 54	73.3± 1.8
26–28	2,518± 53	72.8± 1.8
29–31	2,510± 58	71.5± 1.8
32–34	2,430± 59	69.2± 1.7
35–37	2,421± 63	69.1± 2.2
38–40	2,361± 57	67.7± 1.9
41–43	2,311± 78	66.1± 2.2
44–46	2,274± 60	64.1± 2.3
47–49	2,198± 59	61.9± 3.4
50–52	2,188± 80	59.2± 3.1
53–54	2,140±104	58.3± 3.9
55	2,111±363	54.3± 6.9
56–60	2,051±193	53.5± 6.6
61–65	1,809±125	51.0± 6.1
66–70	1,767±233	43.1± 5.4
71–75	1,624±230	39.6± 9.8
76–80	1,510±376	33.4± 9.8

Index for Average Maximum Ventilatory Capacity and Vital Capacity by Age Group
(Based on 18–20 years old)
(Figures are for one square meter of body surface.)

Age	Vital Capacity (%)	Maximum Ventilatory Capacity (%)
8	61.08	57.43
11–14	73.18	75.97
14–17	87.52	87.45
18–20	100.00	100.00
20–23	95.9	91.64
32–34	90.17	86.39
41–43	86.07	82.52
51–53	81.86	73.91
56–60	76.36	66.79
61–65	67.38	63.67
71–75	60.48	49.44
75–80	56.24	41.70

Physical Effects of Scientific Breathing Therapy

Breathing therapy is one of the most effective health maintenance techniques that the Orient has ever produced. Nevertheless, this method for the preservation of health failed to attract popular attention during the nineteenth Century because of that era's unquestioning acceptance of the values of Western civilization which placed great emphasis upon positive scientific studies. However, medical research, which has made remarkable progress during the past century, has focussed new attention on breathing therapy. What was once regarded as a therapeutic method favored by members of primitive religious sects has now emerged as one of the most authentic Oriental medical techniques and has succeeded in gaining a number of ardent twentieth Century admirers who believe that this Oriental treatment may be a key to the mysteries surrounding human life.

From a physiological point of view, a man could not survive, much the less function, if he were to cease breathing for even ten minutes. Generally speaking, if a person stops breathing for three minutes, he experiences a suffocating sensation. Consequently, as soon as breathing is resumed, the person tends to draw deep breaths as quickly as possible in order to meet the growing oxygen demands of the body. At that point, a person must concentrate on taking deep breaths in order to avoid the immediate threat of asphyxiation; all other matters become secondary. Normally, several minutes of continuous, heavy respiration are required in order for the body to return to normal. In order to understand why human beings instinctively regulate their respiration cycle in order to sustain life, we must focus our investigatory attention on the characteristics of the ordinary respiration cycle.

Oxygen is a gas without color, smell or taste. It constitutes about one-fifth of the earth's atmosphere. For human beings and for most other animate creatures, an interruption in their supply of oxygen for any extended period means death. This is because a continuous supply of oxygen is required in order to provide each cell of the body with the means for converting nutrients into fresh energy resources. In brief, oxygen is one of the most important elements in the maintenance of human body metabolism. This vital supply of oxygen is brought into the body only by means of regular and continuous respiration.

The program of breathing exercise developed in the Orient is aimed at accelerating the supply of oxygen and the elimination of carbon dioxide from the system. Specifically, its pattern of deep respiration is designed to maximize vital capacity by expanding and contracting the lungs. Following the prescribed regimen causes the diaphragm to move to the maximum points in its range, causes the abdominal muscles to intensify the diaphragm's movement in both directions and causes the thorax to expand its capacity to the maximum. The result is a substantial increase in total vital capacity.

The salutary affect of scientific breathing therapy is readily apparent to our medical research team. According to our clinical research, the diaphragms of those

Japanese practicing the deep breathing techniques move to a level 3–4 centimeters below normal during deep breathing exercises. When downward movement of the diaphargm increases by 1 centimeter, the capacity of the thorax increases by 250–300 cubic centimeters, on average. Clinical research indicates that, if diaphragm movement increases in both directions, the capacity of the thorax may increase by as much as 1,000–1,200 cubic centimeters. Each increase in the capacity of the thorax is accompanied by a consequent increase in vital capacity.

The vital capacity of an average man in healthy condition is about 400 cubic centimeters. By consciously breathing in as deeply as is possible and then expelling as much air as is possible from the lungs, an average man can achieve a vital capacity of about 3,500 cubic centimeters. Certain athletes, such as swimmers and marathon runners, and those people who practice breathing exercises show the maximum vital capacity increase to the maximum level of 5,000–8,000 cubic centimeters. The following table sets forth the results of a statistical analysis of the relationship between age and various indicia of physique on the one hand and vital and maximum ventilatory capacities on the other.

Correlation between Vital Capacity and Maximum Ventilatory Capacity and Age and Physique (Height, Weight, Body Surface Area and Pulmonary Vital Capacity)

	Vital Capacity (VC)	Maximum Ventilatory Capacity (MVC)
Age	−0.336	−0.368
Height	+0.471	+0.314
Weight	+0.423	+0.239
Body surface area	+0.525	+0.315
Pulmonary vital capacity		+0.501

Among the factors considered in the foregoing analysis, both VC and MVC were found to have the closest relationship, or highest positive correlation, with body surface area. Age bears a negative correlation to both vital capacity and maximum ventilatory capacity, but the absolute value of the coefficient of correlation between age and maximum ventilatory capacity is higher than the absolute value of the coefficient between age and vital capacity.

In considering these statistics, our research team reached the conclusion that it is appropriate to calculate an average vital capacity and maximum ventilatory capacity, by age, for each square meter of body surface area, since body surface area bears the highest correlation to average VC and MVC. It was determined that each age bracket should span three years. The average vital capacities and maximum ventilatory capacities for each three-year bracket are tabularized on page 23. The figures shown are subject to a 95 percent aberration. The regression equation employed in the calculation of the figures for each age bracket was as follows:

Vital capacity (cc) $= [2{,}875 - (13.8 \times \text{age})] \times$ body surface area (square meters)

The formula for the calculation of body surface area was as follows:

Body surface area $= {}^{40}\sqrt{(\text{weight})^{17}} \times {}^{40}\sqrt{(\text{height})^{29}} \times 72.46$

The formula for the calculation of maximum ventilatory capacity (MVC) was as follows:

MVC (1/min) $= [88.09 - (0.53 \times \text{age})] \times$ body surface area

The foregoing formula was used for all subjects thirty or more years of age. For those less than thirty the following formula was used:

MVC $= 73.3 \times$ body surface area

With respect to the female subjects of our research, their vital capacity appeared to be most closely related to their height (correlation coefficient of 0.463) while their maximum ventilatory capacity bore the closest relationship to their surface of body. As in the case of men, both VC and MVC demonstrated a negative correlation to age. The regression equation employed in the calculation of the VC and MVC figures were as follows:

Vital capacity (cc) $= [2.019 - (10.5 \times \text{age})] \times$ height (in case of Japanese women)
Vital capacity (cc) $= [2.178 - (10.1 \times \text{age})] \times$ height (in case of American women)
Maximum ventilatory capacity (1/min) $= [64.2 - (0.517 \times \text{age})] \times$ body surface area (in case of Japanese women)
Maximum ventilatory capacity (1/min) $= [71.3 - (0.473 \times \text{age})] \times$ body surface area (in case of American women)

Among the many findings which emerged from our clinical research, those which have attracted the greatest attention are the comparative figures on the vital capacity and maximum ventilatory capacity of Japanese and American women. Calculations indicate that American women have greater vital and maximum ventilatory capacities than their Japanese counterparts. Observers in Japan hypothesize that the superior respiratory functions of American women may be attributable to the American style of living which encourages American housewives to engage in hard physical labor. The passive existence of Japanese women in the Japanese community results in inferior physiological respiratory function. Today however, many Japanese women of the younger generation exhibit a markedly improved physical conditions and a consequent improvement in their respiratory functions. This is attributed to the increase in the number of women in professional posts. The newly developed positive role of women in the Japanese community has resulted in an expansion of women's physiological capacities. Medical experts are, therefore, optimistic that the capacities of Japanese women, vis-a-vis those of American women, will show an improvement in the next round of clinical research.

New breathing habits will do much to improve respiratory function. It is most satisfying to observe and confirm the remarkable effects that an intensive program of breathing exercise will have on you and your respiratory functions. However, before embarking on such a program, you must be sure to compare your vital capacity and maximum ventilatory capacity with the average figures for persons of your age and sex. This will provide you with a benchmark from which to measure your progress.

If you are twenty-five years of age or older, and if you find your vital capacity and maximum ventilatory capacity have not decreased, but have not increased either, despite having undertaken a rigorous program of breathing exercise for a period of three years, you should recognize that you have benefited from the exercise. To maintain your physical standards when those of others of like age and sex are in decline is a significant achievement.

Ordinary healthy men breathe approximately eighteen times every minute and during that time take in about 7,500 cubic centimeters of air (normal ventilatory capacity per minute). By comparison, people following a program of breathing exercise breathe approximately six times per minute and have a normal ventilatory capacity per minute of about 12,000 cubic centimeters. Therefore, the deep breathing pattern induced by breathing exercise not only increases normal ventilatory capacity per minute, but also promotes metabolism by substantially increasing the volume of oxygen supplied to and the volume of carbon dioxide extracted from the body. Thus, through regular, deep breathing, a person can increase recuperative powers of the body and make it more resistant to disease by promoting the metabolism and by strengthening the functions of various body organs. By promoting deep breathing, breathing exercise refreshes the body and spirit, invigorates the attitude and stimulates the appetite remarkably.

According to physiological research, there is a particular area of the brain, identified as the respiration center, which control the respiratory functions of the human body. This brain center is located in the occipital region, in an area of the brain known as the medulla oblongata. Obviously, human life can be decisively influenced by the functions of the respiration center. In fact, this respiration center is sometimes referred to as the "center for life." Therefore, if we can promote the functioning of this respiration center by engaging in breathing exercise, it could be said that a fountain of life could be found. Stimulation of the respiration center might first be transmitted to the breathing muscles, causing them to move in a rhythmic pattern. This pattern of regular muscle movement and this mechanism will promote smooth respiratory function which, in turn, will stimulate the respiration center, improving respiratory function and improving physical condition.

Diaphragm movement has a similar effect upon physical and mental condition. Regular diaphragm movements stimulate the solar plexus and stabilize the mental functions. This, in turn, results in a stabilization of the respiration cycle and a consequent stabilization of and improvement in mental and physical condition.

Respiratory rhythm, the rate of respiration, and the regular depth of both expiration and inspiration can be varied in accordance with an individual's will. The main purpose of the breathing exercise is to foster deep, quiet breathing. It is also intended to result in even, measured and refreshing respiration. Those engaged in breathing exercise have an average minute respiration cycle (MRC) of 6, while an average healthy man has an MRC of 18 and this demonstrates the depth and slowness of breathing exercise.

The marked influence of breathing exercise on digestive organs

Digestive organs, such as the oral cavity, the esophagus, the stomach, the duodenum, the large and small intestines and the rectum, perform a number of essential physiological functions, such as the digestion of food and drink and the absorption of nutritive substances for the body. If troubles develop in these digestive organs, stomachache, gastritis, gastric catarrh, gastric ptosis, peptic ulcer, duodenal ulcer, enteritis, intestinal catarrh, and constipation may occur. We can stimulate and massage the various parts of the digestive system, both directly and indirectly, through continuous breathing exercise. Among the various internal organs of the human body, only the diaphragm, separating the thorax from the abdominal cavity, and the abdominal muscles are under the control of the human will, as they are voluntary muscles. The breathing exercise is designed to encourage vertical movement of the diaphragm and contraction and relaxation of the abdominal muscles, with the result that pressure on internal organs within the abdominal cavity is broadly increased. This stimulates their function. Specifically, internal organ function is increased in the following ways:
1. Stimulating, directly and indirectly, stomach, liver, kidneys, intestines and organs, thereby promoting the secretion of digestive enzymes and the others and helping them promote absorption of nutritive substances;
2. Imparting a rhythmic motion to small and large intestines, prompting the digestive process and helping to relieve constipation;
3. Asisting the numerous capillary vessels in the abdominal cavity in the absorption of nutritive substances;
4. Eliminating surplus fat attached to the intestines and the abdominal wall and promoting the excretion of waste materials and
5. Promoting the absorption of fluids and facilitating kidney function.

The performance of breathing exercise may be accompanied by rumbling of the stomach, belching, and the passing of gas. These phenomena indicate the successful achievement of the abdominal movement. As was noted above, continuous exercise of the respiratory organs has a marked and salutary effect on the internal organs of the digestive system.

Remarkable effects of breathing exercise on circulatory system

The blood and the blood vessels of the circulatory system serve as the body's vital transportation facilities. Among the circulatory organs, the aortas and the vena cava play key roles. They are responsible for the transportation of nutritive substances and oxygen to and waste products from all parts of the body. The functions of these organs may not be permitted to stagnate for even a short period. When blood does not circulate properly, muscles, bones, and various cells and organs fail to receive the supply of oxygen and energy resources which they need in order to continue their functions. Similarly, these organs and cells do not discharge the carbon dioxide and other waste substances which have accumulated within them. We must also bear in mind that inadequate blood circulation may also deprive the brain and its cells of oxygen and fresh nutritive substances. This can result in serious acidosis and, permitted to go to extremes, can result in irreversible destruction of the cell structures or even death. In other words, good or bad circulation can seriously affect not only health conditions, but also life itself. Breathing exercises encourage the circulation of blood throughout the body, prevent the accumulation of cholesterol in the blood, and retard the onset of serious illnesses, such as arteriosclerosis and clot.

The consistent breathing exercise also promotes the functions of red and white blood corpuscles. In a maritime analogy, the red and white blood corpuscle are sometimes compared with ships while the blood in the vessels is compared to the stream. The red blood corpuscles are described as merchant ships, carrying oxygen from the heart to all parts of the body and returning carbon dioxide gas, a waste product, from all parts of the body to the heart. The white blood corpuscles, on the other hand, are analogized to battleships which combat problems that develop in tissue cells and bring them under control. Thus, breathing exercise, which promotes the functions of both red and white blood corpuscles, is believed to facilitate both the maintenance of good health and speedy recuperation from various diseases.

Influence of breathing exercise on the nervous system

All of the organs and tissues of the human body and their various functions are under the strict control of the central nervous system. The nervous system is series of plexuses, bound together and administered from a central point, the brain. If a serious problem develops in one of the plexuses, then the parts of the body controlled by the plexus become ill. It is, therefore, necessary to restore balance to the affected nervous plexus before starting the treatment of the affected body parts. In other words, when suffering from a headache or a pain in the foot, it is essential to identify and cure the real cause of problem before proceeding to treat the head or the foot. A person suffering from a toothache will experience serious pain again unless the tooth is fixed by a dentist. A pain killing drug can not do much to restore decayed teeth.

The third main step in breathing exercise is designed to circulate "Ki" (energy) throughout the body. This method stimulates the entire nervous system, both peripheral and central, and is designed to facilitate reflex actions of the nervous system to the stimuli provided by respiration exercise. The exercise is also designed to control the balance between the sympathetic and parasympathetic nervous systems, to place the stimulative and inhibitive functions of various hormones under the strict control of the nervous system and to sensitize the peripheral nerves. By so doing, the physiological functions of the various parts of the body are strengthened and the various systems of the body are restored to a normal condition. The circulation of "Ki" is regarded as similar to those stimuli administered in the practice of acupuncture, moxa treatment and massage. The peripheral nerves are vigorously stimulated, thereby producing a large number of neurons (minimum units for measuring the nervous functions). This promotes the functioning of various internal organs and improves their resistive powers against pathogenic bacteria.

The central nervous system works well to control systematically the functions of various organs. The basic aim of breathing exercise is to stimulate directly the various organs in the body, and to alternatively and repeatedly to strain and relax the nervous system by regularly modifying abdominal pressure through movement of diaphragm and the abdominal muscles.

Relation between respiration and capillary activity

Capillaries expand and contract under the control of the central nervous system. Physiological research has disclosed that a normal man lying quietly drives some 50–60 cubic centimeters of blood into the arterial system with each contraction of the heart. An active man, on the other hand, expels some 80–100 cubic centimeters of blood with each cardiac contraction. Therefore, smooth circulation of blood in the capillaries is absolutely essential in order to lessen strain on the heart.

If the capillaries widen, a larger volume of fresh blood, filled with nutritive resources, is supplied to every part of the body. This facilitates metabolism. Taking long deep breaths permits a widening of the blood vessels and strengthens the expansion and contraction of the capillaries. These results are fully recognized by both Oriental and Western medical science as beneficial consequences of breathing exercise. Blood rises in the face of people undergoing hard physical training or breathing exercise. A person's face also may flush and turn red when he becomes suddenly excited. Conversely, a person may become ashen when he first experiences terrible sensations, uneasiness or worry. A red face is caused by a congestion of blood in the capillaries of the face and paleness is caused by a lack of blood in the capillaries.

The capillary networks of the cerebral cortex, the subcutaneous tissue, the endocrine system, the liver, the lungs, and the intestines are especially dense and support the respective vigorous metabolisms of these key organs. There are some 2,000 capillaries in the subcutaneous tissue per one square millimeter. In a man at rest, only about five of these 2,000 capillaries are actively circulating blood, while in a person undergoing breathing exercise, performing hard labor or participating in sports exercises, all 2,000 capillaries are actively working to circulate blood. These capillaries beat regularly in a certain cycle and this pulse functions like a series of small hearts to circulate blood in the vessels. These small hearts supplement the real heart and can play a very important role in maintaining the body in the best condition.

Hard respiration exercise permits us to activate several millions of capillaries in the body. The facilitation of capillary function in the stomach and duodenum is particularly important for the maintenance of good health. For those who suffer from hypertension or heart disease, the facilitation of capillary function is one way in which to effect a radical cure for these otherwise incurable diseases.

2. Preparation for Breathing Therapy

Points and Purposes of Breathing Therapy

Before practicing breathing therapy, an individual needs to have a definite purpose or goal. A beginner often loses enthusiasm or becomes weary a few minutes after starting the practice. Such a person may give up easily upon encountering an obstacle in the course of the exercise. This failure to persevere may be attributed to a lack of confidence in the therapy or the absence of a definite aim in practicing it. The most desirable way to practice the breathing therapy is to meet all the requirements of the therapy first, divide the practice into small steps, and then master them one by one, with a definite aim, such as recovering from an illness and maintaining regained health. It is also necessary to set a specific time for the daily exercise and to keep it strictly.

Intentional natural breathing

What practitioners in breathing therapy, call "natural breathing" must be "tranquil," "relaxed," "fine" and "equivalent." The respiration of healthy people meets these four requirements naturally. However, the breathing of people who are exhausted, overstrained, in poor health, easily frightened or upset, emotional worried, irritated or impatient is irregular and not normal. For example, breathing of a person in poor health is usually characterized by long expiration and extremely short inspiration or, sometimes, the reverse, that is, long inspiration and extremely short expiration. Neither of these is a normal condition. Continuation of such breathing will worsen the condition. Therefore, the breathing of such people must be controlled intentionally. Once under control, they should endeavor to continue natural breathing.

Natural breathing is unconscious, free from any care and impatience, untiring, easy, continuous and fine. In other words, it is neither long nor short. It should be smooth and well-balanced. When such breathing is attained, a person feels fine, and is no longer bothered by the various obstacles which may occur during the course of breathing therapy exercise. Eventually favorable effects became evident in all parts of the body.

The number and amount of breaths

A normal healthy adult takes an average of 18 breaths per minute. As breathing therapy progresses, the time required for each breath becomes longer. In the advanced stages of breathing therapy, the number of breaths per minute can be reduced to 5 or even 3 or 2. (A Zen priest takes only 2–5 breaths per minute once he is sitting in a Zen manner and has achieved a stable and tranquil state of mind. He can remain in this condition for about thirty minutes.) There are two ways to reduce the rate of respiration. One is to make your breathing fine, and the other to make it deep. In addition to exercising intentional control, you can make your breathing fine by limiting the amount of air inhaled. This can be accomplished by narrowing your nostrils and throat, or by lightly setting your teeth together and touching the tongue to the inside of the gum of the upper jaw. To make your breathing deep, all of the alveoli of the lungs must be activated and the differential between expansion and contraction of the alveoli increased in order that the tidal volume can be increased.

When breathing is fine and deep a longer time is required for each breath, therefore, the number of breaths per minute decreases. However, the total amount of ventilation per minute does not vary very much even if such changes in the breathing pattern occur. For instance, if the minute respiratory cycle is 15 and the tidal volume is 0.5 liters, the total amount of ventilation per minute is 7.5 liters. Assuming that this amount of ventilation per minute is fixed, a five-fold increase in the tidal volume, i.e., an increase to 2.5 liters, means that a total of only 3 respiratory cycles need be taken in a minute. Thus, if the amount of ventilation per minute by a man in normal condition is assumed to be fixed, the tidal volume is inversely proportional to the number of respiratory cycle taken in a minute.

What, then, is a real aim in extending the time required for one breath or increasing the tidal volume? It is to increase the vital capacity, expedite the exchange of carbon dioxide for oxygen and stimulate the metabolism. Further, the fine and deep breathing gives pleasant stimuli to the nasal mucous membrane and activates the function of the parasympathetic nervous system. Deep breathing increases the pressure inside the abdomen and forces surplus blood, stagnating in the internal organs and mesentery, into veins. It also stimulates the solar plexus and helps to tranquilize the mind. Thus, an individual can maintain health and a tranquil state of mind by controlling the respiratory cycle and the tidal volume.

Strength of breath

When you first commence breathing therapy, you are apt to try too hard or to breath too roughly. As a result, you may feel sick or nauseated or have other problems, such as a headache, during the exercise. Medically, this is called "general malaise" and is due to hyperventilation. Therefore, breathing therapy should be carried out patiently, step by step. When you have safely completed the basic stage and feel better than before, you may go on to harder breathing exercise. Such a progression is essential to trouble-free practice of the breathing therapy.

Breathing and blood circulation

Disruption of breathing rhythm and improper respiration may upset blood circulation. The heart sends blood containing a high concentration of carbon dioxide into the lungs and, then, after gas exchange has taken place in the lungs, the heart sends oxygen-rich blood through the aorta to every organ of the body. As can readily be seen, breathing and blood circulation are two closely-related, continuous functions. When they are balanced, your physical rhythm is in order and, when they are unbalanced, it is out of order. Therefore, when undergoing breathing therapy, you must match the rhythm of inspiration and expiration and the length, depth and strength of each breath with the condition of your body. Otherwise, you may experience various problems. As was mentioned above through breathing therapy, you can learn to control the diaphragm and abdominal muscles as well as to increase abdominal muscular pressure. This abdominal pressure forces blood stagnating in the internal organs and the mesentery back into veins, and increases the amount of blood circulating in your body. The increased circulation of blood throughout your body, assisted by the breathing therapy, cures illness and serves as a basis for a healthy body. For people who look pale, suffer from hypotension or anemia, or are adversely affected by the cold, continuous breathing exercise produces remarkable results.

Principles of the Breathing Therapy

There are three basic principles of breathing therapy; they can be summarized as follows:

Body Regulation
Breath Regulation
Mind Regulation

"Body Regulation" means to put your body in order and to have good posture. "Breath Regulation" means to breathe regularly. "Mind Regulation" means to tranquilize your mind and to develop and maintain acute senses. These three are referred to as "Nai San Go" (three inner matches), which can be further explained as follows:

1) matching the mind with the senses;
2) matching the senses with "Ki" (energy); and
3) matching "Ki" with the force.

In Japan (mainly among Buddhists), it has been said from ancient times, that in order to achieve "Samādhi" (concentration of the mind on a single object), one must put the body, the breath and the mind in order. That teaching is consonant with the concept of "Nai San Go."

"Matching the mind with the senses" means to make your ideas accord with your senses. That is, to make the various philosophical and ideological systems of the breathing therapy and the senses you personally have for it overlap each other completely. By thinking in this manner, you come to firmly believe that you will change each part of your body, as expected, through its respective exercise and that eventually you will achieve the original aim. Such a mental attitude is a vital factor to make the breathing therapy effective.

"Ki" is a life energy existing in both the microcosmos (the world inside the body) and the macrocosmos (the world outside the body, including the celestial universe). "Matching the senses with Ki" means to realize "Ki" with the senses. In other words, you can bring "Ki" into play wherever and whenever you want to, through your senses; you can raise "Ki" and lower it as you wish. "Ki" has three aspects. One is the movement of air from nostrils and mouth into lungs, that is, the gas exchange itself. Another is the "Kisoku" which is circulated within the body by the senses. The third aspect of "Ki" is the energy which exists in universal space. When the practice of breathing therapy reaches a certain stage, you can sense that "Ki" is circulating throughout your body in the rhythm of breathing. This state is called, in our technical terms, "Sen Ki Nai Ko" (latent "Ki" moving inside). ·

"Matching Ki with the force" means that each organ in your abdomen relaxes when "Ki" declines, and contracts and becomes tense when "Ki" rises. These contractions and relaxations are generated by breathing and are kept in balance with the movements of the internal organs. If breathing becomes irregular and loses its rhythm, the balance between breathing and the senses collapses, sometimes with serious consequences. Contraction and relaxation of the internal organs are mainly caused by movement of the diaphragm and of the abdominal and back muscles. Since they increase the pressure within the abdomen, the movements of the diaphragm and of the abdominal muscles are regarded as the most important factors in amplifying the effects of the breathing therapy. It is this increase in pressure which is deemed one of the essential conditions, because it stimulates even some involuntary muscles. In a series of functions, the voluntary muscles stimulate the nervous systems and then the nervous systems, in turn, generates reactionary movements in the involuntary muscles.

If you do not concentrate on matching "Ki" with "I" (pronounced "ee," the id) while undertaking breathing exercise, you may not achieve your goal in practicing the therapy, i.e., recovery from illness and maintenance of a healthy body. The exercise will be as futile as shooting without a target.

"I" is a function of the cerebral nerve center. It controls mental and physical functions and works to cure illness on its own by promoting secretion of various hormones and enzymes. The mind and the body can be made healthier as a result. Therefore, "I" must not disregard the guidance of "Ki." Rather, it should strengthen this guidance. In this way, reliable effect can be expected from breathing therapy. In short, the first step in breathing therapy is to let "Ki" circulate throughout your body, following a certain route. The next step is to let "Ki" go to particular parts of the body, depending on what illness you have or which part you want to cure. For example, a person who is suffering from the nephritis leads "Ki" to the kidney, and a person who is trying to strengthen his muscles and body by body-building lets "Ki" go to his wrists, arms, chest, stomach, waist, back, etc., while using a barbell, an iron dumbbell or an expander. During the exercise, the amount of "Ki" to be supplied and the strength of the force must be controlled through precise estimation and measurement thereof by your senses. This is one of the most important factors in the realization of "Ki" with "I."

Side Effects Due to Improper Breathing Exercise and Advice against Them

You may not yet have acquired a correct understanding of Oriental medicine. Some of you, therefore, may offer criticisms such as: "It is an old superstition," "It is not scientific, but religious and philosophical," or "It is not in line with medical principles." Actually, it is the people who make such statements who do not know exactly what is scientific. At any rate, if one continues such criticisms and maintains a cynical attitude toward Oriental medicine, good effects can not be expected from the practice of breathing therapy and the auxiliary exercise. Even worse, such an attitude could cause adverse side effects. Adverse side effects, however, should not be a source of great concern, since most of them are caused by simple errors during the initial stage of the exercise program.

(1) Dizziness and Pain

Some of those who try breathing therapy for the first time feel giddy or experience pain under the roots of the arms or legs, at the waist or in both thighs a few days after starting the exercise. This is caused by suddenly using muscles which have not been used for a long time. One need not worry; such side effects will disappear quickly. Should such pain persist for several weeks, one should consult a physician, as the cause may be something else.

(2) Strong Heart Beat and Fast Pulse

While practicing breathing therapy, your heart may beat wildly, as if dancing, your pulse may quickens, or your limbs may go numb. Unless these phenomena continue for a long time or occur regularly when not exercising, you do not have to worry, as they are temporary reactions. However, if such side effects occur every time you exercise, they are an indication that there is something wrong with your exercise technique; probably, your posture is improper, your breathing is too strong, or your exercise is too long and exhausting. You should check your method carefully and correct what you find to be improper. Further, numbness of the thighs is in most cases, attributable to prolonged standing or sitting. If you experience numbness, you should discontinue the exercise momentarily and do an auxiliary exercise or massage your thighs well to remove the numbness before you start the breathing exercise again.

(3)   Impatience and Tasteless Meals

If you find yourself becoming impatient or if your meals seem tasteless, you probably are breathing improperly, i.e., the length of your inspirations and expirations may be incorrect, or you may be experiencing anxiety about the therapy. If this should occur, you should seek a diversion. Sitting cross-legged or upright and regaining a calm and correct state of mind, or merely taking a walk may help. Further, you should revert to the method of breathing employed during Step I. These actions should be sufficient to eliminate any abnormal reactions.

(4)   Abnormal Feeling on the Skin

You may experience an itching sensation of the skin, as if bitten by an insect. Your hands may become hot, as if warmed over a fire, or alternatively, become cold, as if placed in iced water. When such abnormal feelings occur, you must immediately concentrate on a single object and dismiss all other thoughts from your mind. Since this kind of reaction is incidental to the exercise of the breathing therapy, you need not be concerned.

(5)   Heavy Feeling and Illusion

You may feel as if you are carrying a burden on your shoulders; you may feel as if your arms and legs have shrunk, or you may feel as if your head is swollen and numb. In the worst case, you may feel as if something in your brain is blocking oxygen from reaching the cerebral cells. You may see illusions, have strange thoughts and become extremely emotional. As in (4) above, these phenomena are incidental to the exercise of the breathing therapy and you need not worry. Upon experiencing either of these phenomena, you should immediately concentrate on a single object and dismiss all other thoughts from your mind. With this, the phenomenon should disappear. As you progress with the breathing therapy, they will cease to occur.

(6)   Belching and Rumbling of the Abdomen

In the early stage of the therapy, you may belch a great deal, break wind or notice a rumbling sound inside your abdomen. As was explained earlier, these reactions are attributable to the stimulation of stomach functions which results from the exercise. Although it is very embarrassing to experience such reactions in public, you should not quit your exercise because of it. You can explain the reason to those whom you are with and beg their pardon or you can deliberately schedule your exercise time so as to avoid meeting people while you are still reacting. It is important to continue the exercise until the very end. If you stop halfway, all that you have done will be in vain. The reactions that you may encounter in the course of practicing the therapy are only temporary phenomena.

(7)   Heavy Feeling or Pain in the Stomach and Loosening of the Bowels

A heavy feeling, stomachache and a loosening of the bowels are liable to result if you do the exercise immediately after a meal. Heavy exercise immediately after a meal is not good for the stomach, and the breathing therapy is no exception. You should allow considerable time to elapse between your meal and your exercise.

(8) Nocturnal Emission

Nocturnal emissions are a peculiarly male problem. About ten days after starting the exercise, you may be surprised to find that, in spite of your age, you experience a nocturnal emission. This is not unusual. You may be pleased that the breathing exercise has raised your sexual desire. However, it is not advisable to discharge your revived desire by immediately engaging in sexual intercourse. On the contrary, you are advised to abstain. To prevent nocturnal emissions, you should practice "long exhaling," as in Step I, tighten the anus and rub up and down on both sides of the coccyx with your hands.

As a general rule, you are advised not to exceed the limit of your "Ki" or make a great valsalva suddenly. Otherwise, you will suffer the adverse side effects mentioned above. For a person who is seriously ill or extremely overtired, sudden practice, engaged in a whim, does not improve his condition and may actually worsen it. People with arteriosclerosis, cardiocentesis or hypertension should be especially careful, since such adverse side effects may be dangerous for them. However, too small an amount of "Ki" is ineffective and can neither prevent illness nor eliminate the causes of chronic disease. Consequently, you must evaluate your physical condition before trying to realize "Ki" with "I." The amount of "Ki" is a matter for your sound judgment. Breathing therapy must be performed in a proper manner, it must not be too forceful or too tense. If you do not perform the therapy properly, you may strain yourself, lose your breath, experience numbing of the hands and feet or, even worse, faint. Therefore, you are urged to perform the therapy in accordance with the instructions which follow.

Basic Postures for the Breathing Therapy

When practicing the breathing therapy, you must maintain the proper postures. The three basic postures for this practice are the "erect position," the "sitting position" and the "lateral position." You can in fact, must breathe in any position, lying or sitting. Correct breathing, however, is quite another matter. In order to achieve the desired effects on your mind and body through breathing, you must do it properly; that is, you must assume the indicated postures and forms while performing the exercise. The three basic postures and their variant forms will be discussed below.

Erect position

The "erect position" is, as the name implies, a standing position. It is the easiest, the most healthful and the most creative position among the three, and there are three basic forms for the erect position.

Form 1—Sanen no Katachi (Form of Three Circles)
Since this is the basic form of the erect position, you should learn it thoroughly. Start by standing with your feet together as shown in Fig. 1. Then by moving your left foot away from the right one while counting "one, two" to yourself, assume a standing position with your feet slightly apart. The space between your feet should be approximately equal to your shoulder width. Repeat this exercise until you can consistently place your feet the same distance apart. Next, bend

Fig. 1

Fig. 3

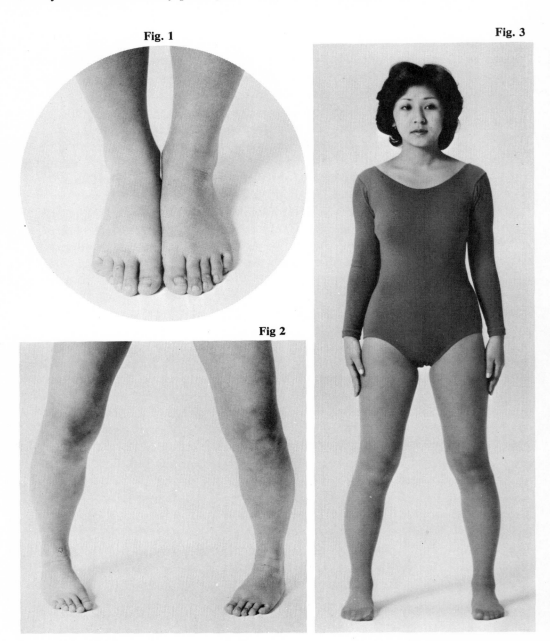

Fig 2

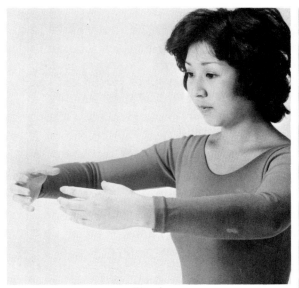

Fig. 4

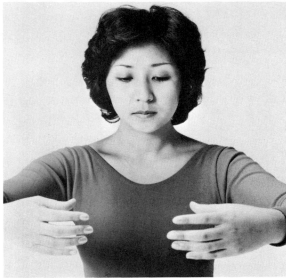

Fig. 5

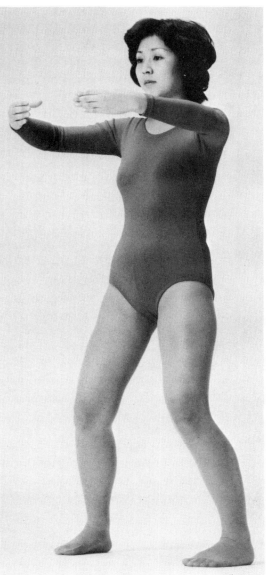

Fig. 6

your knees slightly. At the same time, turn your toes inward as far as possible, forming a half circle as shown in Fig. 2. Straighten your waist, chest and back as in Fig. 3. (Do not be too forceful, i.e., bend backward, straightening them naturally.) When you can do all of these things well, raise your arms to shoulder level, keeping them parallel. Then, bend the elbows to form a circle as shown in Fig. 4. The circle should be as large as possible. This form facilitates expansion of the lungs and enlarges their capacity. The palms of both hands are turned inward, i.e., toward the face. The fingers should be separated, with the tips slightly flexed as in Fig. 5. In this form the fingers will resemble tiger's claws (cupped as if holding a ball very gently). The space between your palms and chest should be about 40 centimeters. Since arm length varies from person to person, the space between palms and chest should be approximately four-fifth of the distance from the shoulder to the wrist. The space between your hands, when making a circle with both of your arms, should be equal to the width of your face. Hold your head up (this symbolizes an unbiased and indomitable spirit) with the neck held straight (Fig. 6). This form is intended to eliminate any unnatural flexion of or pressure on the blood vessels and nerves. Close your eyes half way and look down at a 45 degrees angle. Focus your eyes inward over the tip of your nose or you can concentrate by focussing your sight on some distant object parallel with your half-closed eyes. (The focal point should be a fixed rather than a moving object.) If your eyes are fully open, your mind is subject to distraction by outer stimuli. If you close your eyes completely, however, your senses may become less acute or some other thoughts may intrude and break your concentration. You cannot attain the desired effects in either case. Therefore, half-closing your eyes is the best and easiest way to concentrate and to induce a tranquil state in the cerebrum. (As you may know, the eyes of all Zen priests during Zazen contemplation, and all images of Buddha and Oriental philosophers are half closed.)

The above described form is called "Sanen no Katachi (Form of Three Circles)." The circles are "a circle made by feet," "a circle made by arms" and "a circle made by hands." The purpose of the foot circle is to hold your waist straight and to stabilize your legs so that you stand as if you were a large three deeply rooted in the ground. Both the arm circle and the hand circle are intended to strengthen the breathing function as well as to help transport "Kisoku" to the tips of the fingers. The goal of this form of exercise is to develop and strengthen the muscles of feet, legs, waist, back, arms and hands.

The length of the exercise period should not be long for beginners, three to five minutes at a time, ten minutes at the outside. At first, when the period of time is short, the exercise should be done continuously. This is more effective and facilitates mastery of the form. When you have done a considerable amount of exercise and have become physically fit, you can gradually lengthen the exercise period—eventually up to as much as thirty to sixty minutes. When exercising for an extended period of time, you are advised to do auxiliary exercise (to be explained later) or move your neck from time to time, in order that you can continue the exercise smoothly without becoming fatigued. Eventually you should attempt to reach a point where you exercise twice daily, i.e., in the morning and in the evening, for at least thirty minutes each time. The effects of such exercise are really tremendous.

An advantage of the "Form of Three Circles" is that it permits "Kisoku" to travel simultaneously to the tips of your hands and feet with each expiration, and concentrates it when inhaling in the *Tanden* (solar plexus) where it is condensed.

The condensed "Ki" can be sent by respiration to the top of the head through the spinal cord. This form of "exhaling air roundly, deeply and quietly" is suggestive of a white cloud floating slowly in the sky. It has unfathomable aspects. Professionals describe it as "stepping into a calm river with the weight and force of a mountain, but with an effect on the flow which leaves the river undisturbed." The mind takes a broad view of things, the sensation is heavenly and the "Ki" condensed at the Tanden runs through to the tips of the feet. As mentioned above, if you practice the breathing therapy in this form, your respiration becomes smooth and the "Ki" travels throughout your body. As a result, you feel well and enjoy high spirits all the time.

Form 2—Sangō no Katachi (Form of Three Matches)

This form of exercise follows Form 1. Place one foot about 60 centimeters in front of the other. (The actual distance between the feet should be proportionate to the height of the exerciser, normally, it should be equal to about ⅓ of an individual's height. Further, it does not matter which leg is put forward.) The tip of your lead foot should point straight ahead, while the other foot should be placed at a 30–45 degrees angle from your body direction. (The axes on which your feet are placed should form an ∟-shape.) Bend your front leg, so that the knee is directly above the tip of the foot, and stretch the rear leg gently, so that 70 percent of the weight of your body is placed on the front leg. The waist should be square with the axis of the front foot and held steady. The back held straight. Next, relax your shoulders and raise your hand, on the same side as your front leg, to shoulder height, keeping the palm open and facing upward. The elbow should be bent at an angle of 15–45 degrees and should be situated a little lower than the shoulder (Fig. 7). Raise only your index finger, so that its tip comes to eye level. The rest of the fingers should be bent in the natural manner, i.e., like tiger's claws (Fig. 8). The other hand should be placed so as to rest the back of the wrist on the hip bone. The fingers of this hand also should be bent in a natural curve similar to that of tiger's claws (Fig. 9).

This form is called "Sango no Katachi (Form of Three Matches)." The matches are "a match of the shoulder and the thigh," "a match of the elbow and the knee" and "a match of the hand and the foot." This form is a little more difficult and sophisticated than the "Form of Three Circles" described earlier. Therefore, you must master "Form of Three Circles" thoroughly before advancing to the "Form of Three Matches." If you attempt this form with insufficient preparation, you will be unable to balance your shoulders, elbows, knees, legs, fingertips, waist, etc. The unnatural posture which results will cause pressure on the chest and the abdomen and will strain the muscles. As is true with any program of progressive exercise, you must start with the easiest step and then master subsequent steps one at a time. Otherwise you will not be able to obtain good effects and results.

The main purposes of this "Form of Three Matches" are to intensify concentration of the senses, restore proper function to each organ of the body, lower

Fig. 7

Fig. 8

Fig. 9

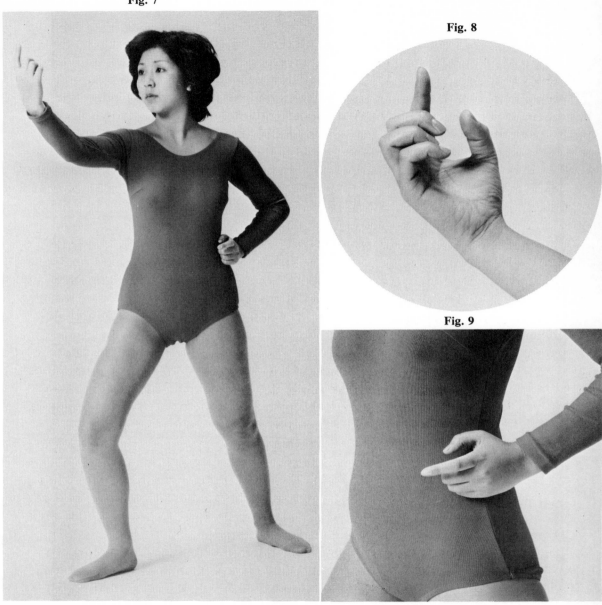

high blood pressure and strengthen the muscles of the shoulders, thighs, elbows, knees, legs, feet and arms. Since the "Form of Three Matches" helps to restore tranquility to the cerebrum, it is a good means of easing nervous tension. Additionally, exercise in this form works to remedy heart disease by lowering high blood pressure. These two are the main effects of Form 2 (Form of Three Matches) in the erect position.

Form 3—Fukko no Katachi (Form of Holding a Tiger Down)

This form is the most difficult of those in the erect position. First, spread your legs laterally, as far as possible, to form a groin angle more than 100 degrees. (As a criterion, your height in this posture should be about four-fifth of what it is when standing in a normal upright position.) The waist should be held steady (Fig. 10). Next, hold your right hand about 10 centimeters above your right knee, while lowering your left arm at an angle of 45 degrees and bending the elbow 90 degrees. Your left hand should be situated in front of your navel. Both palms should be open and face downward. Face the direction toward which

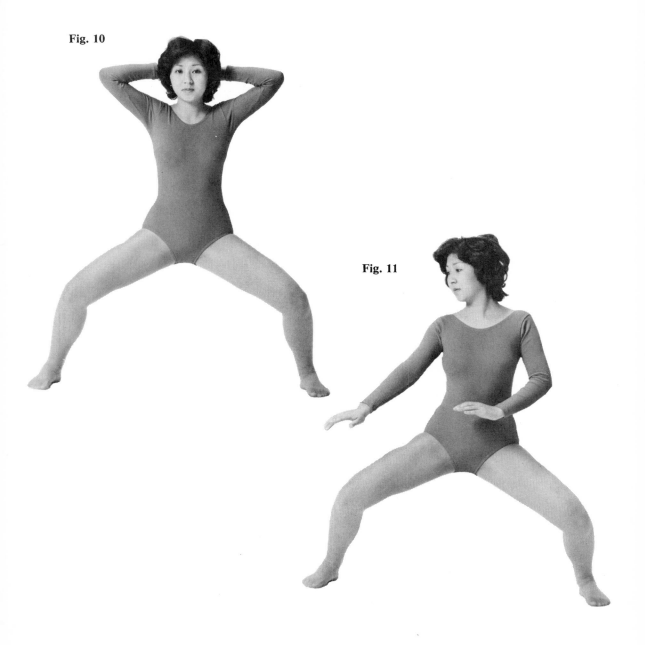

Fig. 10

Fig. 11

your right foot is pointed and close your eyes half way, concentrating your attention on a distant object in front of you. Your head should be upright. This form is called "Fukko no Katachi (Holding a Tiger Down)" as it resembles the posture you might assume if you were holding a tiger's head with your right hand and its back with your left hand. The "Fukko no Katachi" form must be attempted only after you have thoroughly mastered the "Form of Three Circles" and the "Form of Three Matches." If a beginner skips to this form without preparation, his legs may start shaking violently and his thighs may get stiff. Even worse, he may injure his feet, knees, hip joints or muscles. Therefore, you must be very careful when exercising in the "Fukko no Katachi (Holding a Tiger Down)" form.

The purposes of the "Fukko no Katachi" form are to strengthen your arms and legs as well as to build up the muscles of your waist and back. Its practice results in the strengthening of muscles and bones and the remedying of chronic disease. Expiration will give you an exhilarating feeling, similar to that which accompanies the riding of a fine horse or long distance running. Inspiration will impart a sense of power, as if you had fought a tiger down with bare hands. Continued exercise in this form will make you spontaneously spirited and your body will seem to be a wellspring of power.

Merits of the erect position: The reason that the erect position has been discussed first is that, as was noted earlier, it has certain relative merits when compared with the sitting position and the lateral position. These merits may be summed up as follows:

(1)　To order your breathing, you need clean air. Places which meet this requirement are parks, suburbs, fields, woods, riversides, beaches, mountains and the lake. In such places, however, it is inconvenient and unsuitable to exercise in the sitting position or the lateral position. The erect position may be employed in any place.

(2)　The performance of breathing exercise in the erect position does not in the least disturb or put pressure upon your circulatory system. You can, therefore, send "Ki" smoothly to every part and organ of your body. As a result, pleasant stimuli are given to your whole body, in a massage. In this way, the exercise is very effective in curing disease and maintaining health. Though both the sitting and lateral positions are more effective for putting your mind in order and placing it at rest, you cannot expect the effects therefrom to be as good for your entire body as are the effects from the erect position. Further, since stillness and action are closely and cleverly combined in the erect position, it is relatively free of side effects.

(3)　The most difficult aspect of this Oriental breathing therapy is the realization of "Ki" with "I" and permitting the "Ki" to go to the Tanden and then to reach the cerebrum via the spinal cord. To achieve this, you have to become capable of actions such as "tighten the lower abdomen," "grip the ground with the soles of the feet," "tighten the anus" and the like. In this way, "Ki" leads to "Ki" and better effect is obtained.

(4)　To perform the Oriental breathing therapy, you must be especially alert. However, the sitting position and the lateral position are so relaxing that you are apt to fall asleep during the exercise. The realization of "Ki" with the senses is, therefore, quite difficult in these positions. By comparison, it is easier to remain awake in the erect position. "Kisoku" travels throughout your body in the waking state and calms mind and body as well as takes you to the stage where "Ki" leads to "Ki."

(5)　Various auxiliary exercises can be performed in the erect position. Therefore, it permits diversions which enable you to continue exercising for long periods without wearying.

(6)　Since you can raise or lower your arms in the erect position, "Kisoku" moves freely throughout your body and mingles with other "Kisoku" there. It works to expand your lung volume and vital capacity and imparts maximum felicity to the heart and the cerebrum.

(7)　When you have mastered each form of the erect position completely, you can practice the "Three Circles," "Three Matches" and "Fukko" in succession and include auxiliary exercise between them. It is a beautiful flowing movement. (These are the basic forms of *Tai Chi Chuan* exercise.)

Sitting position

The sitting position is divided into two major forms, "Fuzai (sitting with legs folded)" and "Kizai (sitting on a chair)." "Fuzai" is further divided into four forms; "Kekka Fuza (sitting cross-legged)" as in Fig. 12, "Hanka Fuza (sitting

Fig. 12　　　　　　　**Fig. 13**

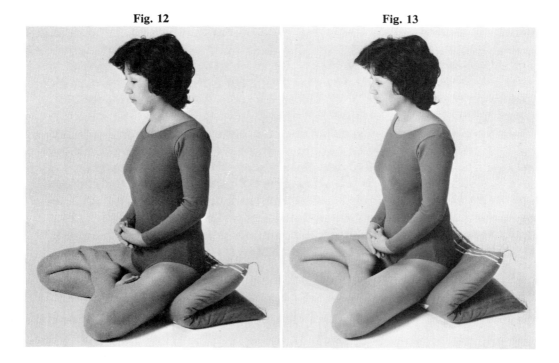

Fig. 14 Fig. 15

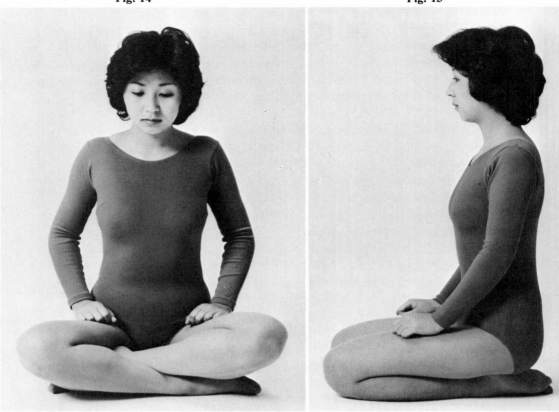

half cross-legged)" as in Fig. 13, "Shizen Anza (natural easy sitting)" as in Fig. 14, and "Seiza (sitting straight)" as in Fig. 15. Each has its own purposes and effects.

Kekka Fuza (Sitting Cross-legged)

This form originates from old Indian Yoga, but is better known, today, as a Zen sitting posture. *Fukanzazengi*, regarded as the Bible of Zen, explains the forms as follows:

> To go into Zen, you should be in a quiet room and neither full nor hungry. Your clothes should be worn in a loose but orderly fashion. Usually, put a thick mat or cushion on the place where you intend to sit; you may sit either cross-legged or half cross-legged. To sit cross-legged, rest your right foot on your left thigh, and rest your left foot on your right thigh. To sit half cross-legged, only put your left foot on your right thigh. Then, rest your right hand on your left foot, and rest your left hand in the palm of your right hand. The tips of both thumbs touch each other. Keep your back straight and do not lean in any direction. Your ears and shoulders should be in one vertical plane, as should be your nose and navel. Touch

your tongue to the upper jaw, and set the teeth and lips together. Keep your eyes open at all times and breathe through your nostrils. When you have put your mind and body in order, expel all of the air out of your lungs. Sway from side to side until you find the right posture; then, hold still. Keep your mind empty without conscious effort.

Although the foregoing description is very difficult to understand, what you should do is to put your right foot on your left thigh, with the sole upward. Then, put your left foot on your right thigh, with the sole upward. Thus, in the "Kekka Fuza," the soles of both feet are turned upward, while both knees press steadily into the cushion. Next, fold the cushion in four, and place it under you. Hold your head, neck and chest upright, and combine both hands in the "IN" manner. Close your eyes half way, and concentrate on some distant point in front of you. Since this form is quite difficult for a beginner, it would be smoother to try it after mastering "Hanka Fuza." Those who are ill or who are frail, after having just recovered from an illness, should not try this form for a while.

Hanka Fuza (Sitting Half Cross-legged)
Put either of your feet on the opposite thigh, turning the sole upward. Then, insert the other foot under the other thigh. The rest of the instructions for "Hanka Fuza" are the same as the instructions for "Kekka Fuza."

Shizen Anza (Natural Easy Sitting)
This is the least desirable form in the sitting position because your folded knees will cause your body to compensate by leaning forward. Your back tends to bend and this puts pressure on the base of the spine and may cause lumbago or the hernia of the intervertebral disc. Therefore, you should be very careful in employing this form.

For all three of these forms, it is best to place a cushion (about 15 centimeters in thickness) under your buttocks for stability. Regardless of the particular form, however, most beginners cannot prevent their feet from going numb while sitting. With practice, it is possible to reach a point where the feet will no longer go numb, no matter how long you continue to sit, even if you sit on a bare floor without cushions. Beginners need not endure the numbness. They may interchange their legs, stand and do some light exercise, or massage their legs from foot to thigh. They can then continue the sitting. A merit of this "Fuza" form is that "Kisoku" flows relatively easily and therefore, can be led to and collected at Tanden. Further, because it is stable, you will be less likely to lose your balance and will be better able to concentrate. Buddhists call this posture "Zengo" and Taoists consider it an essential factor in their "Yōjōkun (method for living daily life)." When exercising in the "Fuza" form, you must try to avoid stiffening of your muscles and bones.

Seiza (Sitting Straight)
This form is closely related to Japanese "Bushido (the code of the warriors)"

Fig. 16

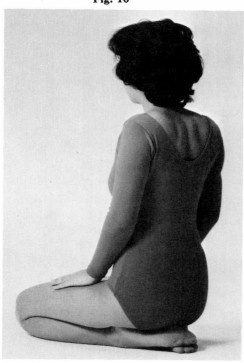

and was developed along with it. Precisely folded legs and a body poised to turn in any direction are among the features not seen in the other sitting positions (Fig. 16).

Keys to seiza
1) Hold your waist upright.
2) Lower the solar plexus.
3) Store nervous energy in the solar plexus, Tanden.

These three keys to "Seiza" will be discussed in detail.

(1) Cross the arches of both feet. Either foot may be placed underneath, but both ankles should touch the floor. Sufficient arch-crossing is the primary element in holding the waist upright. In the early stage of the exercise program, your waist may get sore or numb. As your exercise progresses, however, you will no longer experience such a pain or numbness.

(2) The space between the knees should be about equal to the width of two fists (one fist for women). If the space is too wide, it is the chest which supports the body. This defeats the original purpose of "Seiza."

(3) Thrust your buttocks as far backward as is possible and rest them lightly on your feet.

(4) With your waist upright, sit as if you were attempting to rest your lower abdomen on your knees.

(5) Lean slightly forward, and then release the forces from your chest, shoulders and Tanden. By literally implanting the instruction "to hold your body straight," you may have more of a tendency to draw the chest back and stiffen the shoulders. However, such a posture concentrates force in and stiffens the pit of the stomach. Therefore, you are advised to lean slightly forward and to relax the upper body (above the navel).

(6) Hold your neck high, draw your chin in and turn your face upward. Were you to permit your neck to lean forward, you might be easily distracted by other thoughts and unable to hold power in the lower abdomen.

(7) Tighten both sides of your body slightly and put your left hand on your right one on your thighs, with the arms down along your body.

(8) Close your mouth gently. Set your teeth together lightly and touch your tongue to the palate right behind the upper front teeth.

(9)   Half close your eyes and focus them on a single object in front of you at about 45 degrees below your ordinary line of sight.

As was noted above, "Seiza" is a unique sitting posture developed in conjunction with Japanese martial arts. It is the only sitting posture used in Japanese arts such as Kendō, Judō, Karate, Aikidō, the tea ceremony and flower arrangement. Although there are other sitting forms such as "Hiraza" in Fig. 17, "Tate-hizazuwari" in Figs. 18 and 19 and "Hizakuzushizuwari" in Fig. 20, they will not be explained here since they are unhealthful.

Fig. 17

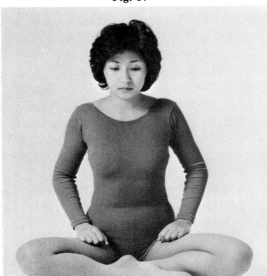

Fig. 18

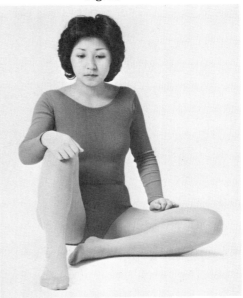

Fig. 19

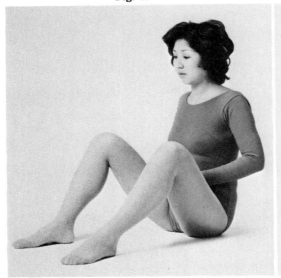

Fig. 20

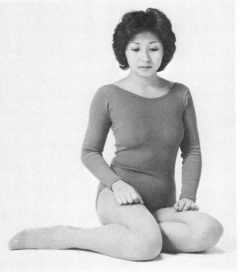

Fig. 21

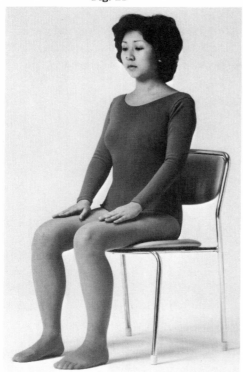

Kizai (Sitting on a Chair)

In this form you sit on a chair of appropriate height (Fig. 21). You position your upper body, i.e., head, neck, chest, etc. as you would in the "Fuzai" form. The space between the knees should be equal to the width of two fists. With the soles of both feet firmly on the floor, your knees should be bent at a right angle. Hold your arms and hands as you would in Fuzai. Close yours eyes half way, also as you would in Fuzai. Since this form is easy, convenient and does not cause numbness even if used for a long time, it is successfully employed by many people, without regard to age, sex or physical conditions. Although the effects from "Kizai" are not as remarkable as those that can be achieved through Fuzai, it is better to continue this form than to give up after only a few days of exercising in the Fuzai form.

Lateral position

There are three forms in the lateral position. They are "Gyoga (lying on one's back)" as in Fig. 22, "Ohga (lying on one's side)" as in Fig. 23, and "Fuga (lying on one's face)" as in Fig. 24.

Gyoga (Lying on One's Back)

Lie on a springless bed (a *Futon* mat on the floor is the best), with your head raised slightly as in Fig. 22. (Depending upon the temperature, you can cover your body with a blanket.) Put your legs together and extend them, with the toes pointing upward. Rest both hands on your lower abdomen, positioning both thumbs on the navel. Close your eyes half way, and look at the tip of your nose. Alternatively, you can concentrate all of your attention by fixing your eyes on one point on the ceiling, 45 degree angles above the horizontal.

Ohga (Lying on One's Side)

This form does not require special inclination of the head as does "Gyoga." (A pillow may be used if you wish.) You just lie down on your side. Keep your body straight, and put the upper leg on the lower one. Bend both knees, but the upper should form a more acute angle than the lower one. You can lie down on which-

Fig. 22

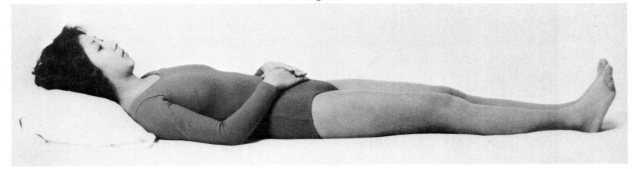

Fig. 23

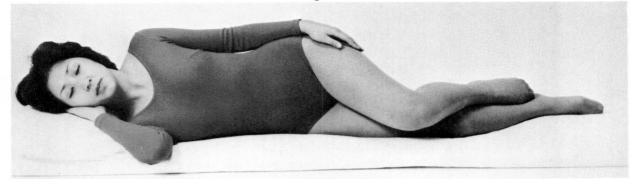

Fig. 24

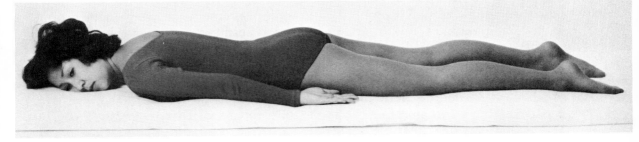

ever side you prefer. However, those who have heart diseases should be careful not to put pressure on the heart by lying on their right side. If you must exercise shortly after a meal, it is best to lie on your right side since that position is supposed to promote and facilitate the digestive functions of the stomach and intestines. If you use a pillow, adjust it so that your face is slightly lower than the back of your head. Place the palm of the hand on the lower side of your body under your head for support. (This helps stabilize the cranial nerves.) Extend the other arm naturally and place it on your thigh. You can concentrate your attention by closing your eyes half way and looking at the tip of your nose, or by starting one point at about angle of 45 degrees from your feet.

Fuga (Lying on One's Face)

Lie face down and extend your legs, spreading them so that the distance between your feet is about 20 centimeters (Fig. 24). Also, extend your arms along your body. Face whichever side you prefer. Close your eyes half way and look at the tip of your nose, or you may stare at a point toward your feet but at an angle of about 45 degrees from the axis of your body. This prone position is suitable for the sick or weak. However, one drawback is that it is conducive to sleep. For those who have chronic diseases of the digestive system, such as gastric ptosis, peptic and duodenal ulcers, an early stage of cholecystitis, nephrolithiasis, pyelitis, constipation, proctoptosis, etc., this prone form is the most effective position.

Seven Steps of Preparatory Exercise for the Breathing Therapy

Compared to Westerners, Japanese still have more opportunities for spontaneous breathing exercise in daily life, e.g., laying *Futons* on a floor and putting them back into a closet, going up and down stairs, carrying heavy things by hand, bowing to greet, sitting straight or cross-legged. Since we repeat these movements often, it is easier for us to perform breathing therapy than it is for Westerners. Abdominal respiration is especially easy for us, Japanese. We do not need to assume a special posture in order to do it, while Westerners, the living in different circumstances, must be firmly committed and must make great efforts in order to master abdominal and other breathing methods. For young Japanese, accustomed to a Westernized style of living way and for Western readers as well, I shall here explain the ancient techniques employed in preparation for the breathing therapy. I shall re-arrange the material to facilitate your understanding. Before starting, blow your nose, go to the toilet room and relieve yourself.

Preparatory Exercise 1

Lie on your back without using a pillow. (You should lie on either a springless bed or a carpeted floor.) Then, rest your left hand on your chest (positioning the little finger on the nipple, in case of a woman, and midway between the pit of the stomach and the throat, in case of a man) and place your right hand on the lower abdomen, positioning the thumb just under the navel (Fig. 25). You are now ready for Preparatory Exercise 1. Close your mouth and inhale deeply and quietly through the nostrils while keeping your left hand pressed down to keep the chest from rising during inspiration. Expand your lower abdomen. Let your right hand remember the feeling of the abdomen swelling. (Your left hand is not just to prevent your chest from moving but to control its movement as well.) Next, purse your lips and exhale, while uttering "Oh" or "U" slowly. At the

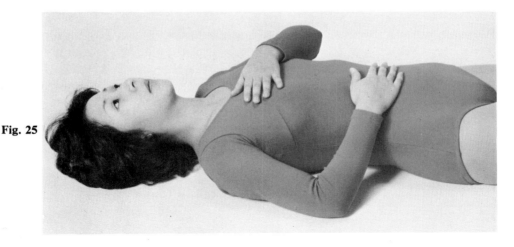

Fig. 25

same time, press your abdomen in the area of the pit of the stomach with your right hand. Your left hand keeps your chest still. After ten repetitions, reverse the positions of both hands and repeat the exercise ten more times. Since each respiration must be done in the same rhythm, ideally you should use a metronome or have a partner beat time with his (or her) hands or count cadence for you. The speed setting of a metronome at ½, simple triple time for inhaling and simple sextuple for exhaling. When you have developed a sense of timing, remove the hands from your chest and abdomen. If you can breathe in the same without the help of your hands, you will have mastered Preparatory Exercise 1.

Preparatory Exercise 2

Lie on your back without using a pillow (the same as in Preparatory Exercise 1). This time, bend both knees upward and touch both heels to your buttocks (Fig. 26). The positions of your hands should be the same as in Preparatory Exercise 1. The breathing method is also the same as in Preparatory Exercise 1. However 20 breaths, instead of 10, should be taken with the hands in each position.

Fig. 26

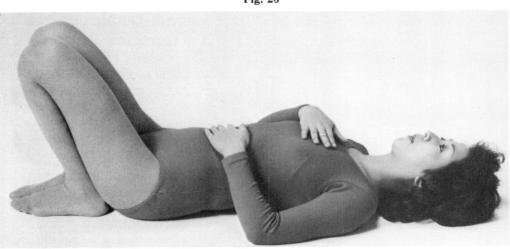

Preparatory Exercise 3

Lie on your side without using a pillow and place the upper leg on top of the lower leg. Then draw your thighs toward your chest, placing your hands in the same position as they were initially in Preparatory Exercise 1 (Fig. 27). Take 10 breaths, then change sides, reverse the positions of the hands and repeat the exercise.

Fig. 27

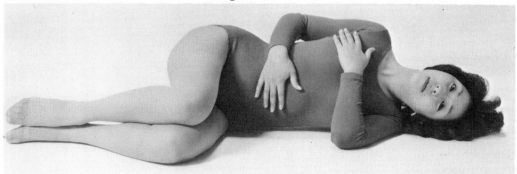

Preparatory Exercise 4

Raise the foot of a bed about 25 centimeters. Lie down, face-up, with your head at the lower end of the bed (without a pillow). Put a weight of about 500 grams on your lower abdomen, and take 50 breaths in the same manner as you did in Preparatory Exercise 1 (Figs. 28 and 29). Add an additional 500 grams every three days until the total weight being used is 2,500 grams. When you have become comfortable with the 2,500 grams weight on your abdomen, you may begin to extend the exercise time gradually to a maximum of thirty minutes.

Preparatory Exercise 5

A cloth 30 centimeters wide and 180 centimeters long is required for this exercise. First, sit erect on a chair. Then, fold the cloth in half to a width of 15 centimeters, and wind it around your waist—more specifically, the area between the pit of your stomach and your navel—and cross it in front of the pit of your stomach. Leaving some length at each end, grasp the cloth firmly (Fig. 30). Now you are ready. Loosen the cloth simultaneously with each inspiration, and tighten it simultaneously with each expiration (Fig. 31). The breathing method should be the same as in Preparatory Exercise 1. This exercise coordinates three movements, i.e., breathing, the movement of the hands and movement of the abdomen. If you do the exercise correctly, you should be unable to tell whether your breathing is loosening the cloth or whether the tightening of the cloth is promoting your breathing. All movement should be in perfect unity. When you reach this stage, you will have developed the ability to intentionally control your breathing. Do this exercise in three postures, i.e., sitting on a chair, standing and walking, taking

Fig. 28

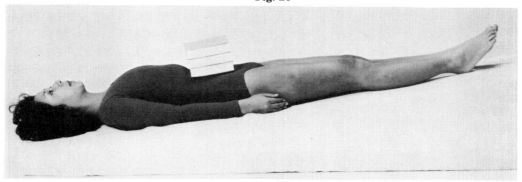

Fig. 29

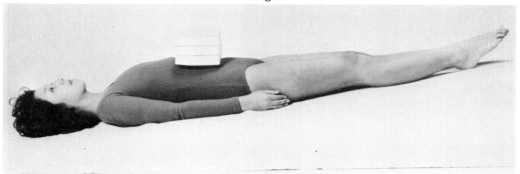

Fig. 30

Fig. 31

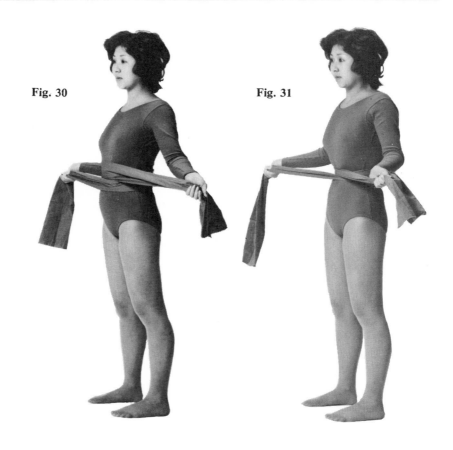

30 breaths in each posture. In the walking posture, however, you must learn to coordinate your breathing and your walking. Begin by inhaling while placing your left foot forward. Then, while exhaling, take three steps forward. At first, it is extremely difficult to coordinate all of these movements, i.e., breathing and moving your hands and abdomen as well as your feet, simultaneously. You should be patient, however. Once you master this exercise, you can practice abdominal respiration wherever and whenever you wish.

Fig. 32

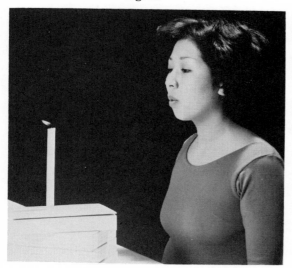

Preparatory Exercise 6

Unlike Preparatory Exercises 1–5 above, this exercise is intended to strengthen exhaling muscles and increase abdominal pressure. A 30 centimeters candle and a stand for adjustment of the candle height (a stack of books will do) are required. Set the candle on a table and light it. The height of the flame should be adjusted so that it is at the same level as your mouth when you are seated on a chair. Place the candle so that it is 15 centimeters from your mouth. Purse your lips and slowly blow the flame by abdominal expiration. Do not extinguish the flame, but bend it forward with a deliberate, slow and strong stream of air. Try to maintain the same flame angle from the time when you start blowing until you exhale all of the air from your lungs. Perform this exercise for five minutes everyday, extending the distance between your mouth and the candle by 5 centimeters per day. The eventual goal is to be able to bend the flame from a distance of 100 centimeters. When you have mastered this, do the same exercise from a standing position. (Don't lean forward during this exercise.) If, for some reason, you cannot use a candle, suspend a paper tape 1.5–2.0 centimeters in width and 30 centimeters in length so that it hangs in front of your mouth. Blow it in the same manner as you would blow a candle. If neither a candle nor a paper tape can be used, just imagine a candle with red flame on the empty table and pursing your lips, blow at it. The strength of the air stream should be controlled not by your mouth but by adjusting the abdominal muscles so that the force exerted thereby is constant.

Preparatory Exercise 7

You need two wide mouth 2-liter bottles, two 20 centimeters lengths of rubber hose, one ∩-shaped glass pipe (30 centimeters × 40 centimeters × 30 centi-

Fig. 33

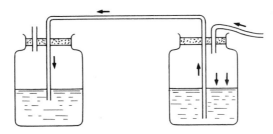

meters) and two corks (which fit the bottle mouths and which have two holes each, one for a rubber hose and the other for a glass pipe: Fig. 33). Attach a paper, graduated in centimeters, to the outer surface of one bottle. Pour 2,000 cubic centimeters of water red or blue colored into it. Connect the two bottles with the glass pipe. Each end of the glass pipe should be 0.5 centimeters above the bottom of its respective bottle. Make the quantity of the water in each of the two bottles equal (i.e., halve the water in the first bottle). At first, do this exercise sitting on a chair. Hold one of the rubber hoses in your mouth and breathe with the abdominal muscles. Lower the water level with 1 centimeter by one expiration. Then, clamp the rubber hose with your teeth, and inhale air through the nostrils. Hold your breath for three seconds. Then, lower the water level another 1 centimeter. Repeat this five times lowering the water level by 5 centimeters in total. (In other words, that much water is transferred from one bottle into the other.) On the second day of this exercise, lower the water level by 2 centimeters with each expiration, transferring 10 centimeters of water (800 cubic centimeters) into the other bottle in a total of five expirations. Increase the quantity of water transferred by one expiration by 1 centimeter every day until you can lower the water level by 5 centimeters in one expiration, that is, 25 centimeters (2,000 cubic centimeters) in a total of five expirations. In this exercise, you must not move your chest. Use only the abdominal muscles so that you can master perfect abdominal respiration. Also, be careful not to lean while exercising forward. If big-mouth bottles are not available, fill a basin with water, put your face into it and pursing your lips, slowly exhale air. Another alternative is to fill a bath tub with water, hold a rubber hose in your mouth and exhale air into the water. The hose should be lowered in the water gradually as your exercise progresses.

Tension and Relaxation Exercise

Tension and relaxation: these are essential to practice of breathing therapy. Although no visible force is exerted on the body, internal systems are continuously contracting and relaxing as part of the breathing process. The tension mentioned here is not valsalva breath holding, but rather, natural breathing which produces calm force slowly and steadily. The continual contraction and relaxation is like a massage to your body, it quickens the entire blood circulation and eventually brings health. It is therefore very important to learn the principles of this contraction and relaxation process and to understand them completely.

First of all, you must learn the importance of relaxation. Many people pay attention only to contraction and are ignorant of the importance of relaxation. The first step in breathing exercise is to relax the muscles. Having your muscles and mind relaxed is essential to effective practice of the breathing therapy.

The exercise begins with air expiration. First, relax your shoulders, arms, hands, feet, abdomen and then gradually all other muscles until your entire body is completely free of tension. Then, relax your mind and liberate your spirit. Expiration must be performed slowly and quietly in order to relax the muscles of your shoulders, arms and hands gradually, in that order. Relaxing the muscles of your shoulders, neck and arms facilitates blood circulation in those areas and gradually relieves you of fatigue. In this way, you can prevent your body from becoming exhausted; if you are not exhausted, you are not easily troubled; and if you are not troubled, your mind is calm and stable. With that state of mind, you feel well prepared to cope with any new difficulty which might arise. Thus, through a feed-back effect, body rhythm continually improves. Relaxation occurs when respiration gets into a proper rhythm and the more the muscles relax, the more harmonious the respiration becomes. In other words, the better your control of "Ki," the more your muscles will relax. Since most beginners cannot relax all of their muscles with one expiration do not attempt the impossible. You should try not to inhale excessively. Rather than relaxing erratically, it is more important not to shake the shoulder muscles or make the muscles tense intentionally. With the second expiration, try to relax the muscles gradually, and from around the fifth expiration, attempt to do it in earnest. When your relaxation technique has become smooth (i.e., expiration is smooth and uninterrupted and you can relax the muscles without erratic movement) begin practicing inspiration exercise. Once you have mastered the technique of relaxing by exhaling completely, try increasing tension by inhaling a little at a time.

In the initial stages of breathing therapy, you must master, through repeated exercises, the ability to alternate between relaxation and contraction as you inhale and exhale. The object is to be able to cause your abdomen to contract and relax intentionally. For instance, when you lift something heavy or want to do something forceful with your hands or feet, it is useless to concentrate force in your face or chest. You concentrate force in your lower abdomen, cause it to contract and carry out the job. Also, when you do chin-ups on an iron bar, the concentration of force and the contraction of muscles takes place in your lower abdomen. Abdominal contraction is the key to the entire exercise. Exercise to relax and contract the abdominal muscles also lowers high blood pressure, prevents cerebral vascular disorders and eases nervous tension. If you maintain the relaxed condition of your abdomen for some time after the conclusion of the relaxing exercise, the degree of relaxation increases and its effects become greater. After having practiced this exercise several times, you will develop a slow rhythmical movement in your abdomen with each breath. This natural rhythmical movement pushes blood stagnating in the abdomen into veins and facilitates blood circulation. If, at this moment, you concentrate all of your attention on your abdominal movement, you would clearly sense that the blood is circulating throughout your body. It is at this moment that we breathing therapists say "the delivery of 'Ki' has been realized."

Side Effects of Being Tense and Slack

Side effects could be serious, especially for those with a history of neurasthenia or hypertension. These people, therefore, must be very careful in performing this exercise. Because people suffering from such problems tend to become easily excited by even insignificant stimuli, they may unconsciously shift from "just holding a breath at the point of changing inhaling to exhaling" to "valsalva breath holding," with a resulting rush of blood to the head. The cerebrum then becomes excessively stimulated and this may lead to sleeplessness or even cerebral apoplexy. Consequently, people who are suffering from neurasthenia or hypertension, and those showing such tendencies, are warned not to generate unnecessary tension by completely failing to exhale at all.

Concentration of Mind

When you practice breathing therapy for the first time, you cannot avoid exerting unnecessary force and making rough and spastic movements. Concentration of your mind is even more difficult and it is unlikely that you will be able to achieve this all at once. First, you must become as mentally relaxed as is possible and attain a calm state of mind. Then, gradually, without disturbing that calmness, concentrate your attention below the navel, on Tanden. Start breathing slowly, trying to prevent your attention from being distracted from Tanden. Then, gather "Ki" at Tanden below the navel. This harmonizes the heart and blood and stabilizes the mind. We call it "falling into the state of mental pleasure."

A concrete method for concentrating the mind is to use "Sūsokukan (the breath counting system)." Another way is "Mokushō-hō (recitation method)." This involves the recitation of some rhythmical and mentally stabilizing verse, such as a passage of a sutra. Though there are some other devices to improve concentration, I will first describe the method for attaining such state intentionally. To concentrate the mind is to direct all of your attention to a single object. Reading, studying, taking a test, calculating mentally, and most other intellectual work requires intentional concentration of your attention. You must focus on a single object without permitting yourself to be distracted by anything else. The Zen guidebook has this to say on the subject: "The place to rest your mind is in principle the palm of your hand. But when you feel depressed, it should be placed on the top of your head or between the eyebrows. Or when your concentration is loose, put it at Tanden, and when you are exhilarated, position it on your foot."

The first step in developing concentration is to determine where your mind should be focussed. The object of your concentration can be anything anywhere. For instance, a distant view, the light of a floor stand lamp, a cigarette lighter left on the floor, your aching stomach, or anything else. However, the object of your concentration need not be an object or part of your body. It can be an ideological abstraction, a worry or a pain. What is important, however, is that your concentration not be forced.

It is said, in Zen, that "not worrying is an ailment" and that "enlightenment comes from doubts." When your mind is occupied by a worry or an anxiety, you should concentrate on the problem and resolve it positively. The concentration required is the same as that which you try to attain by counting your breaths or by silently reciting verses.

When all attention is concentrated on a single object, breathing spontaneously becomes ordered. (For example, imagine that you are aiming a rifle at a target.) When breathing is ordered, the spirit is stable. Therefore, focus your attention on Tanden and concentrate so that your breathing becomes deep and quiet and your spirit becomes more stable. Your mind should be completely clear at this stage. If you can maintain this condition for an extended period, you will be relieved of all worries and anxieties and will enjoy limitless pleasure. This is the time when "the mind" and "Ki" become one in perfect harmony. The effects of this on the health of both the mind and the body are remarkable. If you suffer from a disease, recovery will be accelerated regardless of its nature.

The second step for concentration of the mind is to bring all your attention to one without consciousness. While exercising the intentional concentration mentioned above, you are to gradually acquire an ability to harmonize the body with the mind without intentional efforts for the concentration. We call this state "Sanmai (luxury or pleasure)."

Focussing on Tanden

A word almost indispensable to any discussion of Oriental martial arts, medicine or fitness techniques is "Tanden" or "Tanden below the navel." Opinion as to its location is divided. According to one old book, the position of Tanden is in front of the kidneys, below the stomach, above the "Tsubo" named "Kangen (CV-4)" and 9 centimeters below the navel. Another old book on medicine describes Tanden as follows: above it is the stomach, below it is "Kangen (CV-4)," behind it are the kidneys and in front of it is the navel. Actually, the location of Tanden is in the center of the abdomen, about 4 centimeters below the navel. Additionally, another book says that the center of Tanden is the crossing point of "Okimyaku (one of the eight meridians and a line from the Hyakue (GV-20) of the top of the head to Ein (CV-1)" and "Ohmyaku (one of the eight meridians and a line circling the waist)." These lines resemble the Chinese character "田 (den)," after which the position is named "Tanden." Although there are various opinions, predominant opinion at present is that Tanden is below the navel. (Put both thumbs together on the navel, and join index and middle fingers of both hands below it. You will observe a heart-shaped space between your hands. The inside of this heart shaped area is Tanden.)

In breathing therapy, all senses must be led to Tanden during breathing in order to make the cerebrum stop thinking temporarily. That is, attention is concentrated on Tanden. When your breathing becomes stable and rhythmical, let the intentional concentration on Tanden become relaxed and permit your imagination to take its own course. Although you may be unaware, you will be filled with a new vigor which will strengthen the kidneys and activate the functions of the internal organs. In breathing therapy, this is called "Kennō, Kenjin" and is considered as one of the basic requirements for healing any ailment.

Next, there is a saying that "attention protects Tanden." This means that extraneous thoughts should be dismissed from the consciousness and the state of "Nai San Go, tension and relaxation" should be sought through the "one mind, one attention (concentration of the mind on a single object)" method. In other words, concentrate your attention on a single object at first, and gain control of "Ki" so that it may be transported down throughout your body. Then create the condition of "no hearing and no seeing" and maintain it. At this stage, you can be serene, selfless and unselfish.

Generally speaking, it is very difficult to attain this state at the beginning of your exercise. However, when, through continuous exercise, you become better able to focus your attention on Tanden, extraneous thoughts will disappear from your consciousness and the nerve center of the cerebrum will calm itself. People who have difficulty in accomplishing this are continually annoyed by extraneous thoughts during the exercise and become troubled by such distractions and their concentration deteriorates further. This is because they try to continue the exercise with their heads only which results in a break-away of "Ki" and an impoverishment of the cerebrum. This is totally inconsistent with the aim of resting the mind. The rhythm and balance of the breathing will collapse and the effects of the exercise on ailments and/or health will be gone.

Why does the concentration of attention on Tanden bring "Kennō, Kenjin"? In Tanden, i.e., in the area below the navel, there is a gathering of many autonomic nerves called the solar plexus. When these nerves are activated, blood vessels and capillaries in the area of the abdomen up as high as the waist are stimulated, thus facilitating the absorbtion of waste and the efficient discharge thereof through organs such as the liver, the kidneys and the colons. Detoxification of body waste and noxious substances by the liver and the kidneys is especially facilitated. Swift removal of noxious substance speeds recovery from fatigue and helps produce new energy to cope with new work. This applies not only to the body but also to the spirit. Therefore, you will be balanced both physically and mentally. Having been relieved of fretfulness and restlessness, you will feel calm and stable. For those who are still unable to concentrate on Tanden through the breathing method or the concentration of attention, I will offer the following advice:

Method 1:   Prepare a cloth 30 centimeters wide and 180 centimeters long, similar to that which was used in Preparatory Exercise 5 of the seven Preparatory Exercises to the breathing therapy mentioned before. At first, fold the cloth in two and tightly wind it all around your waist from the pit of your stomach to above the navel. The key is to draw in your upper abdomen when you wind it. Next, sit cross-legged and settle down completely. Bend your upper body forward and lower so that you are facing the navel and the lower abdomen. Then, expand your swollen lower abdomen further, by distending it with air, and stroke it in a circular pattern with either or both of your hands. Though this is not an attractive pose, you should practice it, for the sake of your health, without being ashamed. In Japan, this cloth is called "Enju-obi (belt for a long life)" and regarded as a key to a long life.

Method 2:   For this method also, use a cloth 30 centimeters wide and 180 centimeters long. Fold the cloth in two and wind it tightly around the body from below the navel down to the pubic bone, i.e., over the Tanden. Draw in your lower abdomen winding, and bind it tightly with the cloth. Then, straighten yourself, form "Seiza" and keep quiet. Inhale air through the nostrils and send it to the lower abdomen. Holding pressure there, exhale the air. Repeat this breathing. Directing force into the abdomen is not unique to the breathing therapy. Everybody used to do so when *kimono* were worn daily in Japan. It is still quite important and necessary, especially in Japanese dancing, flower arrangement, the tea ceremony, martial arts, etc.

Here, I will tell you about an interesting experiment. Though this is sometimes formally referred to as "Goltz's Experiment," we call it "mesmerism by a street showman." First, catch a chicken, turn it upward and then press its abdomen sharply. The chicken goes faint instantly. The result is the same in the case of other small animals. This is because the plexus of the parasympathetic nerves in the lower abdomen is excited by pressure and, when excited, it checks the function of the heart, reduces pulse rate and lowers blood pressure. Thus, a temporary sleeping condition occurs, as if the animal were mesmerized. Oriental people in ancient times knew from experience that putting force into the abdomen or winding a sash tightly around it produces transition of the senses, and used the technique in daily life to gain or maintain health.

3. *Practice of Breathing Methods*

The Breathing Method That Has Been Handed Down Generation to Generation in the Orient

The Oriental people in the past have had a view of nature containing divine and human factors, as have many ancient peoples, and have had a pantheistic view of nature in which deity, human beings and nature are internally united.

As a general term for nature in the Orient, the word for "heaven" is used. "Heaven" takes on a meaning not only of the sky overhead and all natural phenomena but also the deity lives therein. For this reason have been performed the many ceremonies worshipping "heaven." Although "heaven" is a deity which has no explicit divinity, it is integrated into nature and since nature has the character of a deity, it follows that human beings obey nature. So-called "Sokuten principle" (obedience to heaven) originated from this.

"Sokuten" means to conform to the laws of heaven. The law of heaven includes not only the cherishing and cultivation of all things under the sun but also the movements of the sun, moon and stars, the alternation of the four seasons—spring, summer, autumn and winter—and all other natural phenomena.

In the Orient obedience to nature is the materialization of life itself. Since sowing and harvesting crops and all other things are conducted in natural rhythms, the people are inclined respect nature as a deity by taking the natural order as absolute. However, human beings are to not only merely obey nature but to seek unification with nature. This is the philosophy of unification of human beings with heaven.

As stated above, the element that constitutes the nature and deity which comprise "heaven" is "Ki." "Ki" is a gaseous substance composed of all things including heaven and earth, that is, it indicates a general gaseous body. It should be noted that this principle can be seen set forth in the *Nihon Shoki*:

> There is first the false sky. The universe is born in the false sky. "Ki" is created in the universe. "Ki" has weight. That which is light and transparent thinly overhangs to become "heaven," and that which is heavy and turbid sinks and solidifies into the earth.
>
> The light and transparent "Ki" tends to congregate but the heavy and turbid "Ki" is late in agglutinating. Therefore, "heaven" was created first and then there came the earth.
>
> "Ki" in "heaven" becomes "Yōki," and "Ki" on the ground becomes "Yinki." Of these two "Ki," the pure forms constitute the four seasons of

spring, summer, autumn and winter, and the "Ki" welling out therefrom constitutes the myriad things of creation.

When only "Yōki" combines, it becomes fire. Pure "fire" becomes the sun. When only "Yinki" combines, it becomes water. Pure "water" becomes the moon. "Ki" overflowing from the sun and the moon then becomes the moon. "Ki" overflowing from the sun and the moon then becomes the stars. Thus "Ki" is a gaseous substance forming not only heaven, earth, the sun, the moon and the stars but also all the things of creation. At the same time it is also the fundamental element constituting the mind and body of human beings.

Humans absorb the "Ki" of heaven and earth through respiration. To respire is to nourish body and mind by taking in the "Ki" of heaven and earth. "Ki" in some cases accordingly means respiration itself. "Ki" in "breath" respiration has been ascribed as the source of human life. "Ki" in this sense is, so to speak, the energy of life force itself.

The "Ki" accumulated in the body through respiration builds up the human body and mind. As is indicated by such terms as "temperant" (kishō), "vitality" (kiryoku), "courage" (yūki), "inborn disposition" (kirin), and "intrepidity" (kihaku), "Ki" is a fundamental factor constituting our hearts and minds.

In the ancient Orient, the organs of the body were called the five "Zō" organs and six "Fu" organs. Ancient people held that men's bodies were composed of the "Zō" section and the "Fu" section and that the two sections are the fundamental elements of life activity, performing important roles such as respiration, digestion, and circulation.

Of these, respiration was thought of in two major aspects. Air in respiration, that is, "Ki" (the open air) is composed of "inspiration," which goes down to the liver and kidneys through the nose and the spleen, and of "expiration" which goes up from the heart to the lungs and outside through the mouth. "Ki" is a general term for life energy.

When solid food enters the stomach through the esophagus, it is digested by digestive juice from the spleen, and the effective components changed into the "Ki of the five tastes." The "Ki of the five tastes" is gathered in the spleen where it is mixed with water.

When the "Ki of the five tastes" mixes with water, it creates blood, it was thought. And whenever expiration or inspiration passes through the spleen, it pushes out the blood. The blood pushed by expiration or inspiration was considered to advance into the veins 3 sun (about 9 centimeters) a time. In this manner, expiration, inspiration and circulation are carried out in close mutual interdependence.

"Ki" example A of the ascetic hermits

Human beings live in the open air and "Ki" should therefore be replete in the body. All things in the universe live by "Ki." If a man circulates "Ki" well in his body, he can fill his body effectively with "Ki" and extend its benefits to all parts.

As for the external effects, "Ki" will ward off various evils and work for stabilization of the mind. However, the general public takes "Ki" as an everyday matter. Although they perform respiration, from beginning to end it is mere respiration to them because they do not know the value of "Ki."

How can we perform effective respiration by which "Ki" can be taken into the body?

One method to make the body healthy and strong is to breath out the old air in the body and take in fresh air. If the "Ki" in the body becomes weak, it cannot make up for decline by itself and medicine must be taken as well.

A lack of "Ki" in the body can be responsible for a coughing fit or difficulty in breathing after expending too much strength in running about at a fast pace.

A lack of blood can be responsible for pale complexion, dry skin, weak pulse, or flabby skin. If "Ki" and blood run short, not only physical defects but mental weakness as well may eventuate. A man in such a state is said to face difficulty in maintaining life without taking herbal decoctions.

If "Ki" is taken into the depths of the body and well utilized, supernatural forces can inhere to a person inasmuch as "Ki" is the fundamental energy of life. Specifically, it will cure disease, build up the body to resist disease, speedily halt bleeding, build up a strong mind to overcome fear and a strong body to withstand thirst or hunger.

The secret of long life is the so-called "Taisoku" (fetal breathing). It is a method of breathing like that of a fetus in the womb.

First of all, you take "Ki" into yourself slowly through the nose by breathing, and contain the "Ki" inside your body. You must then count in your mind up to the number 120 and then respirate the breath through your mouth slowly. When you practice this method of breathing, you must achieve a state of silence paying utmost attention to not making any noise in taking "Ki" into your body through expiration and inspiration. When this breathing is being practiced, you have to try to take inasmuch "Ki" as possible in inspiration and to keep "outgoing Ki" in expiration to the minimum. This is to keep the body full of "Ki" by blocking its escape.

When this method of breathing is practiced, you can put a swan's feather between your nose and mouth, and try to breathe without moving the feather. You have to repeat the breathing practice until you count to 1,000 in you mind. With success in counting up to 1,000, an old man may reach the stage of a man in the prime of manhood in several months by thus rejuvenating day by day. However, "Taisoku" should be conducted in the period of "Seiki" between twelve o'clock midnight and noon.

"Ki" example B of the ascetic hermits

A man met a wise man who looked as if he were about 50 years old and had a noble and clear mind different from ordinary men. Accordingly the man questioned him about it. The wise man called himself "An old man." The man asked him in a respectful humble manner how he also could become such a wise man. The key to long life which he received was this "Fukkihō (the method of taking in 'Ki')."

The secret of long life is, first of all, to lie on the right side of your body. After your legs are drawn in, you must face east by putting your head to the south. You then close your fist with your thumb inside. (This is fetal, similar to a fetus in the womb.) The tongue should lightly touch the lower jaw in order to contain the "Ki" in your body. Further, you have to swallow the "Ki." In this manner, you swallow "Ki" seven times and breathe out once.

Then chew the "Ki" seven times, fourteen times or twenty-one times and breathe it out once. After adjusting the breath (to comfortable breathing), you practice as mentioned before, and repeat forty times without straining. The important point is not to strain to chew the "Ki" but to do it smoothly. When you breathe out, do it slowly and quietly by puckering up your mouth.

After you practice the method of breathing without error, lie on your back and draw up your knees to contain the "Ki" in your abdomen, then clench your fists lightly and put them to both sides and slightly below the navel fourteen times or thirty-one times. If you do this, your body will be filled with "Ki." Then, breathe out once slowly. After finishing the practice, you must adjust your breathing again. If you adjust your breathing again after the practice and then repeat, it will have more effect.

Then after taking a deep breath with rapid intake, try to contain "Ki" inside the body by doing practice breathing fourteen times or twenty-one times before breathing out one time. After that, stroke your abdomen to adjust the condition of the whole body before taking a break. You will find you perspire profusely and your whole body will feel warm, that is, you are now full of "Ki." All the joints in your body become activated.

Practicing the method for ten years without fail, a declining body will be rejuvenated like that of a young man and the mind will be clear so that you too may become a wise man.

"Ki" example C of the ascetic hermits

The body has an inseparable relationship with breathing. A healthy person lives a reasonable life everyday without being aware of it. However, those who wish to practice considerable moderation should first try to adjust their bodies by cultivating "Ki." Following is a brief lesson on how to cultivate "Ki."

Lie down everyday at a set time and put all thoughts out of your mind, then take a breath through the nose quietly and breathe it out through your mouth in the manner so that no noise can be heard from either the inspiration or expiration. Then clench your fist (with the thumb inside, fold the index finger first, then the middle finger, the ring finger and little finger in that order).

Holding your breath, send it around and through your body without straining at it and continue until your plantae perspire. When they do, breathe out quietly through your mouth.

Don't feel satisfied when you succeed in doing this once. You must repeat again and again. If you practice more than hundred times a day, you will achieve significant effects. If you are troubled with body heating and perspiration, breathe out slowly puckering your mouth.

By practicing this method of breathing several thousand times, you can build up a healthy body without the aid of medicine. Together with the method of breathing, quaffing reasonable amounts of alcohol in the morning and evening will potentiate the effective results achieved.

If you have gastrointestinal weaknesses, sip a glass of water (about 200 cubic centimeters) in the morning when you wake up (water not too cold but of skin temperature is best). If you do this, the stomach and intestines will be cleared and let "Ki" easily pass through. This simple everyday method should be highly valued for making moderation and nurturing possible. You will know and see the results naturally without others having to tell you.

This method of breathing can also be performed sitting on a chair comfortably. First, you sit back in your chair and loosen clothing and belt to make yourself comfortable. Then shut your eyes, touch the tongue lightly inside the upper jaw and breathe out slowly taking time.

At the beginning inspiration and expiration will be rough enough to be audible to a person next to you. Gradually it will narrow. The sound of breathing will become quite small after you practice the breathing fifteen or sixteen times. By that time, you may fell some pain or itchiness, but you must realize that this is because your breathing is expelling the undesirable from you.

When you have performed your breathing seventy times counting from the first rough respiration, you must repeat from the beginning, that is, the first rough breathing, and repeat this many times.

A physician of the times asked a wise man whether breathing should not be rough. He also asked when, after so much effort, breathing had become calm, one should return to the first rough breathing.

A wise man replied that good breathing as mentioned before, is fetal breathing, but if I toid the average man about such breathing methods from the beginning, he might believe that the smaller the breath is, the better the result and, as a result, many would become as inactive as if they were sick. To avoid this, the best way is to have them repeat the pattern of breathing starting from strong and rough breathing to gradually calmer and quieter breathing.

Those who master the breathing pattern may engage in the method of breathing mentioned at the beginning. In short, the objective is to have them learn how to deliberately control their respiration by performing it in an orderly manner with suitable stimulation.

"Ki" example D of the ascetic hermits

The wise man or master maintains that the key to long life is to simply practice the method of "Ki," cherish the deity (that is, to ensure the long-term retention of a sound mind by strengthening the principle of unity of character from disregarding perils to one's life and the possibility of mental and physical senility) and to breathe properly. Accordingly, you must always breathe out "the old" from your body and take in "the new." If a man breathes through his nose, cultivates the deity and always keeps this principle, he will surely enjoy a long life.

When breathing is performed very quietly through the nose as if there is no saliva in the mouth and respiration is made longer and thinner than usual, the five "Zō" organs (lung, heart, spleen, liver and kidney) will always be healthy and function properly. If the five "Zō" organs are safe, "Ki" will be cultivated smoothly within your body. This is because disease cannot remain in your body when the various organs are working well. Accordingly, you feel that whatever you eat or drink, tastes good, visual and hearing abilities are enhanced and that wisdom is gained. You feel that your body is light and full of energy and that you have dynamic physical strength and will. Everyone should live for a long time. The question is, however, how does one acquire a practical way of doing so?

During the day, the time between midnight and noon (from 24:00 hours to 12:00 hours) is called "Seiki" and between noon and midnight (from 12:00 hours to 24:00 hours), "Shiki." This way of thinking is a unique Oriental philosophy in which man and the universe are unified, Oriental philosophers consider that the universe breathes in the same way as man and, like the human being, when it breathes out the old and takes in the new, the universe is said to breathe out old "Ki" and take in new "Ki."

It was thought that the universe breathed once a day, that is, inspiration was thought to involve live "Ki," "Seiki" hour, and respiration dead "Ki," "Shiki" hour. Accordingly, all things in the universe must take in fresh air as much as possible during the "Seiki" hour in order to ensure its good circulation inside your body. If this is done during the "Shiki" hour, it will be bad for you because this is the time when every type of waste material has been expelled into the universal space. Accordingly, the breathing method to take in "Ki" must not be done outside the "Seiki" hour because it is only in the "Seiki" hour that "enlivening spirits" will be found on the earth and in the universe.

To master the method of obtaining the "Seiki," you lie on your back, shut your eyes and clench your fists firmly (with your thumb inside and four other fingers outside). You breathe mentally counting up to 200 and then breathe out through the nose. If this is done every day with a gradual increase in the number counted to, your mind and five "Zō" organs become progressively safer from becoming diseased.

When you take "Ki" into your body, and the number you count up to reaches 250, your heart, brain and abdomen will always be filled with "Ki." Later, when the number you count to reaches 300, your brain will be clear, your eyes bright and your body become healthy and free of disease.

If so, it is said that a man will be able to live for as long as he wishes.

Outline of the Breathing Therapy

This introduction to the primary step of the breathing therapy is compiled to let people know of its effectiveness.

The breathing therapy's roots can be traced back into practice of Yoga in Hinduism and the Oriental philosophy characterized by the unique combination of Buddhism, Confucianism, Taoism, and Japanese Shintoism.

I have confirmed the various influences of this therapy by closely studying each of the exercise patterns which it involves for the past fifteen years. This intensive study thus gives me a firm ground to give proof of the effectiveness of the therapy.

In the particular study, two undergraduate university students, one graduate university student, one housewife, one single woman, and I took part as subjects. Five Zen monks, all of whom belong to the Sōdō Sect, were also chosen as controls in the experiment.

In experimenting the nine basic respiration exercises that this therapy involves, nine basic items were closely investigated to gather information on the reactions to each of these exercises. The items under investigation were: the minute respiration cycle; the amount of ventilation (per minute); tidal volume; oxygen consumption (per minute); carbon dioxide metabolism (per minute); the respiratory quotient; pressure on the abdominal muscles, electroencephalogram; and electrocardiogram.

A similar investigation was conducted among the five monks under controlled situations. The results of the study are described at the end of the comments made on each respiratory exercise.

The significance of deep breathing

To adapt the program of the breathing therapy according to the individual's physical condition is vital. This will bring the best results in building up a strong physique to resist illnesses and diseases.

Diligent training is also necessary to reap best results in regulating the functions of the body, breath, and the mind. The therapy identifies the functions of both the body and the mind through undergoing several rounds of breathing exercises. Therefore, the building up of sound mind and body is its main aim.

People are apt to think that breathing is carried out unconsciously. After all, one breathes automatically, even when one is asleep, they say. This belief, however, is wrong. White-collar workers who live in polluted and crowded areas of big metropolitan cities throughout this country especially should become aware of this as soon as possible.

The main reason for why they should is simple. In older days, people lived out in the open. Barefoot, they ran around open land to chasing wild animals and game. They rode on the backs of wild horses, tilled paddy fields, chopped fire-woods, and raised loud voices. These people began to prepare for the various difficulties that they were starting to confront. Then, they became familiar with the breathing exercises for the training of both mind and body. This led them to naturally perform certain breathing exercises best suited to their respective physical conditions.

Modern men usually reach adulthood without undergoing many training experiences. They are therefore accustomed to the typical thoracic breathing. But this method of thoracic breathing is a shallow form of breathing which utilizes only the lungs. Particularly, only the upper parts of the lungs are used in such a way that the respiration cycle becomes irregular. Therefore, intensive training is necessary to strengthen the functions of the lungs and the bronchia prior to undergoing the difficult breathing exercises in this therapy.

What is the best way to strengthen the functions of the lungs? First, keep an upright posture when undergoing this therapy. For example, sit upright in a chair as is done in the Western tradition (Fig. 34).

Get a chair and sit deeply into the seat with both feet fixed on the floor. If you feel that the chair is too high, adjust the height by placing some books or a form of platform under the feet. If you feel that the height is too low, put cushions under your seat. Keep your knees at the same height as that of your waist while sitting on the chair. Leave a space of two fists between the knees. (In case of females, a space of one fist is sufficient.)

Stretch up vertically in the position and draw in your chin. Keep your eyes low at a 45 degrees angle. Raise your arms to the level of your shoulders, and curve them inward slowly. Pull both hands toward the chest until the hands touch the chest. Both shoulder blades must turn toward each other, backbone as the hinge when the elbows are pulled backward. After the elbows and the arms are drawn back to their limits, place both hands on the thighs. Keep your upper body straight with the shoulder blades thrust a little outward from the back of the chair.

When in an upright posture, keep the following points in mind (Fig. 35): Both feet are placed apart shoulder width. The knees are slightly bent to balance the body. Throw out the chest to keep the upper body straight even when sitting erectly on a chair. Keep the shoulder blades tightly turned toward each other and the backbone must be at the center. Draw in your chin, and gaze at a 45 degrees angle. Keep your eyes half opened. Relax facial muscles and loosen the jaws at first. Then tighten and relax them in accordance with the regular respiration cycle. When relaxing the muscles, the tip of tongue should touch the front part of the under jaw, near the root of the lower teeth. Keep the upper and lower sets of teeth apart so that your lips are naturally closed. For those people with irreg-ular sets of teeth, that the jaws and the mouth be positioned as naturally as possible is what matters. Strain is felt less greatly when the exercises involved in

Fig. 35

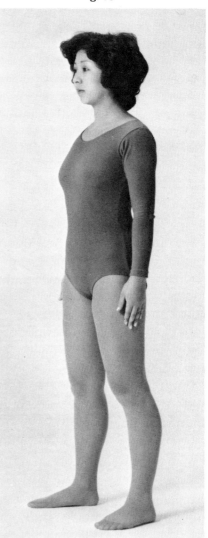

Fig. 34

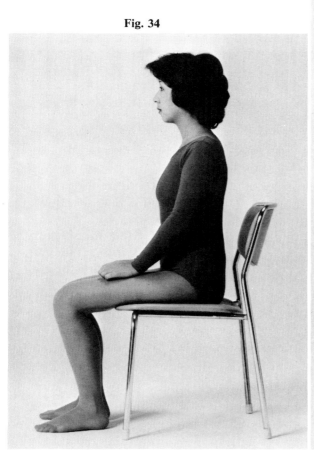

the breathing therapy are conducted in such a posture, because no major frictions will occur when breathing through the nose or through the mouth. The more relaxed the oral and nasal cavities the easier it is for one to carry out the exercise.

Breathing from the nose

Before going into an explanation of the nine basic respiration exercises, certain preliminary points regarding respiration should be studied. The main reasons for this are as follows:

It is necessary to breathe through the nose because the interior of its cavity must be consistently moist. One reason that the nostrils are covered with hair is to warm, to an extent, the cold air breathed into the nasal cavity as well as to moisturize the dry air collected from outside while filtering it of bacteria and germs before it reaches the lungs. This is the reason why impurities and mucus gather here.

It is said that more dirt clogs the nasal cavities of those who are live in urban areas where air is polluted with smog and particles of dust than of those people inhabiting suburban areas where the air is less polluted.

The nasal mucus of those people who work in environments filled with gaseous substances and irritating odors is often found to have resulted in serious inflammations. In some cases, inner walls of nasal cavities are found to have been decomposed in some form or another.

Such phenomena prove that the nasal cavity prevents hazardous substances from entering into the body through the respiratory process. A number of capillary vessels run through the interior wall of the nasal cavity, in a fashion similar to a hot water supply system, the nasal cavity is like a heater of air from outside, adjusting it to the temperature of the body. The adjusted air is then sent down to the bronchia and the lungs through the process of inhaling.

The mucus of the nasal cavity produces an enzyme called lysozyme which works to kill germs contained in the air which have entered the body through the respiratory process. Now, you may understand the importance of nasal breathing in the light of the physiological aspects mentioned above.

Furthermore, the flow of air gives the mucus in the nasal cavity rhythmical stimulus which in turn stimulates the central nervous system, which also helps stabilize the mental well-being of men.

Importance of extended exhaling

Generally speaking, extending the exhaling process brings about considerable improvements in the physical aspects of men. This is because it gets rid of old and stagnant air from the body. The extended exhaling also remarkably reduces the density of carbon dioxide contained in the blood. To strengthen the functions of the diaphragm and the muscles used in exhaling is very important. Holding the breath is the basis of the making of a strong man.

What can people think of while holding their breath? Do they think of their worries at work, family troubles, financial troubles, or sexual difficulties? Actually, they do not or rather cannot, for they have no time for such things. Instead, they are totally immersed in the desire to start normal breathing in order to escape from a feeling of suffocation. This desire transcends the hardships of daily living. Such state of mind and the stimulus given to the nervous plexus lay a foundation for the release of mental stresses believed to be the cause of various illnesses.

Breath-holding is divided into two types: negative pressure and positive pressure. Both stimulate the lung's alveoli, which is believed to trigger the start of a new respiratory cycle. They also give stimulus to the abdominal cavity, thereby influencing various internal organs of the body.

Among the nine basic breathing exercises in the therapy, Steps 7, 8 and 9 are each a combination of both breathing and physical training, in the latter of which bending and stretching of the body are emphasized. These exercises are designed to quicken the circulation of the blood and the rhythmical aspect of breathing. Furthermore, it works to strengthen the abdominal muscles in order to increase the activities of the digestive organs.

Relationship between breathing and the abdominal pressure

We have already learned that the purpose of the breathing exercises is not only to promote air exchange in and out of the body but also to introduce a form of stimulus to the abdominal region. This stimulus, resulting in increased abdominal pressure through the strengthened muscles, drives extra blood, stagnant around the mesentery, into the veins. How exactly should one impose pressure on the lower abdominal region effectively?

Before dropping off to sleep each night, stretch your legs out fully on the bed. Be sure that the body is relaxed, and concentrate. Inhale from the nose deeply, and hold the air for a while, and, while pushing it toward the lower abdominal region, exhale gradually next. When inhaling, count one; when exhaling count two. In this way, count your breaths as it is believed to be a very effective measure in calming the mental state and in being quietly inspired.

Counting your breaths means concentrating your mind on the respiratory activities. Count the number from one to four consecutively, and then return to one again. Repeat this for about 500 rounds each night.

The following points must be followed in breath counting exercises:

1) Inhale from the nose and try to push air down toward the lower abdomen from the chest and the upper abdominal region. Keep remember to expand the abdomen a little and make it slightly hard. Do not, however, try to conduct valsalva breath holding by closing the throat in an attempt to harden the abdominal part. This rushes blood up to the head, face and the neck regions. When inhaling, take as much time as is naturally possible.

2) After inhaling from the nose, take a pause for a few seconds. After holding the breath, exhale gradually.

3) Exhale air as slowly as possible, from the bottom of the lower abdominal region through the upper abdomen and the chest, and through the nose. When exhaling, remember to lower the abdomen a little bit more than usual and pull its muscles in.

4) Having exhaled from the nose, hold your breath counting from one to four. Pause between each count.

5) Repeat the exercise. Generally, four respiration cycles are completed per minute. Therefore, conduct this exercise for 15–30 minutes. This means a total

of 60–100 rounds of inhaling and exhaling are to be completed before one is allowed to rest. Make it a rule to conduct three sets of this 15–30 minute exercise per day. This means that 300 rounds of the respiration exercise are to be conducted every day.

6)   One may stand upright, sit on a chair, or stretch out full length on the floor to perform this exercise. One may even walk or sit on the floor while doing it. Once you are accustomed to this exercise, you can conduct it while doing needlework in the dining room or while cooking in the kitchen. It is also possible to be practicing it while engaged in office work or reading. One thing to remember regarding your posture when carrying out the exercise, though, is to keep it erect in one way or another. Also, if walking, walk at a stable pace with the length of each step equaling the length of your shoulder. Keep the upper body straight. Furthermore, if sitting on a chair, sit in deeply and stretch your backbone upright. Hold up the head and fit it there. Set your eyes on a certain object. Join your hands and set them on the knee; using them to count when sitting is suggested.

When standing, place both arms flat on the sides of the body. If lying on your back on the floor, thrust both feet out and place both hands on the underbelly.

For beginners, it is necessary to keep close track of whether the lower abdominal muscles are being put to full use. Therefore, place both hands inside the belt.

7)   It is vital that the upper body be relaxed while undergoing this exercise. The muscles in the neck, chest, shoulders, face, head, and hands are all be totally loose. The waist, the legs and the abdominal region, however, must be concentrated on fully. Unless the points mentioned above are paid attention to, especially by beginners, a rush of the blood to the head or dizziness may occur.

Continuous pressure is to be imposed on the lower abdominal part when undergoing this exercise. How can this pressure prove effective?

Physical pressure on the abdomen is caused by contraction and tension imposed on the diaphragm, the abdominal muscles, the waist muscles, and the backbone. This pressure gradually concentrates in the central part of the body, between the fourth and fifth lumbars and on the median line. This pressure activates movements, as well as the muscles in the waist and the abdomen. The intensity of this pressure is in proportion to the relaxation of the movement and muscles in the chest, shoulder, hands, neck, head, and face. In particular, the abdominal pressure stimulates the sensation of motion in the heels and the big toes of the feet.

This is caused by the activation of the vagus, which consists of the pelvic ganglion, the sympathetic ganglion, and the inferior mesenteric ganglion at the center, stimulates the central autonomic nervous system, and promotes a sense of balance and coordination throughout the body. The activation also works to intensify the coordinated activities of the autonomic nervous system.

Accordingly, the cerebrum, which directs the body's sense of balance, is stimulated with the introduction of pressure on the abdomen. Furthermore, the pressure excites the sensory area of the brain proper through thalamic radiation, which is brought on by the stimulation of the cerebrum. The pressure thus leads to total activation of the sensory aspects of the brain.

The total activation of the perception in turn leads to coordination of senses, vital in memory functions. At the same time, simultaneous awakening of the central autonomic nervous system enriches emotional functions. The network of nerves controlling movement works to solidify the will when the system is totally coordinated throughout the body. Therefore, it is said that abdominal pressure gives physiological grounds for the purification of the will.

Interrelationship between Breathing and Abdominal Pressure

What is the relationship between breathing and abdominal pressure? In broad terms, they are as closely related to one other as two wheels on an axis. Respiratory training automatically means intensive exercises involving the abdominal pressure.

The main aspects of breathing exercises are as follows: The time spent in exhaling must be more than that spent when inhaling. Each respiratory cycle must be carried out fully and calmly. Pressure both inhaling and exhaling must be conducted rhythmically. Breathing should be conducted through the nose. When respiration is involved, the various muscles in the chest as well as the diaphragm and abdomen all take part in the process. Specifically, among the muscles involved in the respiration process are external intercostal muscles and internal intercostal muscles.

Among the auxiliary muscles taking part in the process of inhaling are anterior, medial, and posterior scalenus muscles, serratus posterior superior muscles, major and minor pectoral muscles, sternocleidomastoid muscles, levator scapulae muscles, and rhomboideus muscles. The muscles in the diaphragm take part in the process of exhaling. When these muscles are moved in coordination with the movements of the diaphragm in order to intensify each respiratory process, vital capacity of functions is increased, thereby improving the alveoli of the lung and hastening the circulation of both blood and lymph.

Remember that the abdominal pressure must be exerted in upright postures, be it when one is standing, sitting or lying down. While undergoing the exercises, the walls of the chest are to be lowered slightly, and strength must be exerted in the waist region. The upper body must not lean forward or backward nor should it bend sideways. (Thrusting the hips out and tightening the anus helps.)

The main part of the therapy is to strengthen the abdominal muscles during the process of exhaling. With all your might, exert efforts to strengthen the muscles while exhaling slowly from the nose. Keep the anus tight. The abdominal muscles can be worked out to maximum limits in this way.

Nine Basic Methods for Breathing Exercise

Type 1. Rhythmical breathing method

This breathing method, called purification breathing, is designed to be carried out in preparation for the nine breathing methods to be introduced hereafter.

In the first stage, inhale and exhale through the nose. Do this five times. On the final expiration, purse your lips and, with full force, expel all air from the lungs. After this, hold your breath while counting "one, two, and three . . . ." Having finished the counting, exhale the air through the nose by relaxing all breathing muscles. Then, take as much air as possible in one slow draught and return to the first stage.

Some may find it helpful to make a tape recording of the instructions for this exercise, and to play it while they are practicing. For example, you might try placing the following instructions on tape: Inhale through the nose, in a slow draught, making a sound like "soo." Exhale all air through the nose with full strength, making a sound like "foon." Inhale smoothly through the nose in one draught, "soo." Exhale all air from lungs with full strength, "foon." Inhale through the nose into lungs in one slow draught, "soo." Exhale through the nose naturally, "foon." Inhale smoothly in a slow draught, "soo." Exhale all air from the lungs with full strength, "foon." Inhale through the nose into the lungs in one slow draught, "soo." Exhale all air from the lungs through the nose naturally, "foon." Inhale through the nose into lungs naturally and slowly, "soo." Exhale all air from the lungs through the nose with full strength, "foon." Inhale through the nose into the lungs naturally in one draught, "soo." Pursing your lips, exhale all air from the lungs in a slow draught, "foon."

While exhaling, take care to contract the abdomen and attempt to draw the diaphragm upward. Exhale and then hold your breath. Pausing for a while without breathing. Next, relax your body and begin counting, "one, two and three . . . " for about five seconds. Then, inhale carefully through the nose into the lungs "soo," and return to the first stage.

It will take about 20–30 seconds to complete each respiration. Keep in mind the fact that air must be expelled from the lungs as forcefully as possible. Each inspiration/expiration should be steady and uninterrupted. As a result, you should be able to complete only about two or three respirations per minute. It is desirable to practice this breathing method rythmically, and imagining, while practicing it, that you are sawing wood. This breathing exercise should be pleasant and relaxing. You must remember, however, to exhale more vigorously than you inhale.

Manual for this breathing exercise: Ordinarily, men take 14–17 breaths per minute and have a total ventilatory volume of some 12–16 liters per minute so that reckoning backward, it takes only about 4.0 seconds for each respiration—2.5 seconds for an inspiration and 1.5 seconds for an expiration. These figures are rough estimations of the average speed for each act of respiration. The principal objective of this type of breathing is simply to exchange air in the lungs. Therefore, it is essentially thoracic breathing with a relatively small amount of pressure being contributed by abdominal respiration.

References: The following chart shows average comparative heart rate and alpha wave rate figures (recorded by electroencephalogram) for an individual during and immediately after this breathing exercise:

	Heart rate	Appearance rate of alpha wave	
		Parietal	Occipital
During exercise (A)	80.0	44.89	75.67
After exercise (B)	82.0	43.81	78.09
(A)−(B)	−1.2	+1.08	−2.42

As indicated in the above chart, the number of heart beats per minute observed after the exercise increased by 1.2 over the rate which was observed during the exercise. After the exercise, the alpha wave rate in the parietal region decreased by 1.08 percent over the rate registered during the exercise, while an increase of 2.42 percent over the rate observed during the exercise was recorded in the occipital region. Compared with the other nine basic breathing exercises, the alpha wave rate in the parietal region ranks fourth while that in the occipital region ranks fifth.

Fluctuations in minute respiration cycle (MRC), minute ventilation (MV), tidal volume (TV), minute oxygen consumption (MO_2), minute carbon dioxide metabolism (MCO_2) and respiratory quotient (RQ) are given in the following chart:

Subject	Minute Respiration Cycle	Minute Ventilation (l)	Tidal Volume (l)	Minute Oxygen Consumption	Minute Carbon Dioxide Metabolism	Respiratory Quotient
A	14.5	16.7	1.1	0.318	0.397	1.25
B	15.0	10.3	0.68	0.200	0.260	1.30
C	17.0	24.9	1.46	0.308	0.498	1.25
Mean	15.5	17.3	1.116	0.305	0.385	1.262

$$RQ \text{ (Respiratory quotient)} = \frac{\text{Carbon dioxide metabolism}}{\text{Oxygen consumption}}$$

Things to be remembered: First, keep your posture erect. Remember to thrust your chest forward, but be careful to keep your chin pulled. Then, inhale through the nose. (If any particular instructions are given, then follow them.) All respiration should be done rhythmically. Take as much air as possible in one draught, then exhale as much air as possible from lungs. (But do not overexert yourself.) Bear in mind also that you should limit yourself to 3–5 minutes for each round of breathing exercise and be careful not to exceed the five minute limit. Make it a rule to perform this type of breathing exercise at least three times per day.

Type 2. Prolonged breathing method

Keep your posture erect and practice rhythmical breathing, in the manner descirbed in Type 1, three times. It should take about one minute. Pursing your lips, exhale all air from the lungs in an attempt to empty them, "foon." While exhaling, gradually contract your belly and try to raise your diaphragm as high as possible. After exhaling, hold your breath and relax. Then count quietly, "one, two, three . . . " for five seconds. Slowly inhale the air into the lungs, while counting "one, two, three." Then hold your breath, while keeping your posture natural and count "one, two." Next exhale through the nose, while counting "one, two, three." Hei, hold your breath, while keeping your posture natural, and count "one, two." Slowly inhale air into the lungs, while counting "one, two, three, four." Then, hold your breath, while keeping your posture natural and count "one, two." Next, exhale air from the lungs, while counting "one, two, three, four." Hei, hold your breath, while keeping your posture natural, and count, "one, two." Slowly inhale air into the lungs, while counting "one, two, three, four, five." Hei, hold your breath, while keeping your posture natural, and count "one, two." Exhale air through the nose, while counting "one, two, three, four, five." Hei, hold your breath, while keeping your posture natural, and count "one, two." Inhale through the nose, while counting "one, two, three, four, five, six." Hei, hold your breath, while keeping your posture natural, and count "one, two." Exhale through the nose, while counting "one, two, three, four, five, six." Hei, hold your breath, while keeping your posture natural, and count "one, two." Inhale through the nose, while counting slowly "one, two, three, four, five, six, and seven." Hei, hold your breath, while keeping your posture natural, and count "one, two." Exhale through the nose, while counting "one, two, three, four, five, six, seven." Hei, hold your breath and quietly count "one, two." Slowly inhale through the nose, while counting "one, two, three, four, five, six." Hei, hold your breath, while keeping your posture relaxed, and count "one, two." Exhale through the nose, while counting "one, two, three, four, five, six." Hei, hold your breath, while keeping your posture relaxed, and count "one, two." Inhale through the nose, while counting "one, two, three, four, five." Hei, hold your breath, while keeping your posture natural, and count "one, two." Exhale through the nose, while counting "one, two, three, four, five." Hei, hold your breath, while keeping your posture relaxed, and count "one, two." Inhale slowly through the nose, while counting "one, two, three, four." Hei, hold your breath, while keeping your posture natural, and count "one, two." Exhale through the nose, while counting "one, two, three, four." Hei, hold your breath, while keeping your posture natural, and count "one, two." Inhale through the nose slowly, while counting "one, two, three." Hei, hold your breath, while keeping your posture natural, and count "one, two." Exhale through the nose, while counting "one, two, three."

Now, repeat the first stage, gradually increasing the count from three to seven. Perform the breathing exercise five times, increasing the number counted to in each repetition from three to four to five to six and, finally to seven. Then, reverse the process, decreasing the number counted to in each repetition from seven to six to five to four to three, while performing the breathing exercise five times. It will take about one minute, on average, to perform one repetition of this exercise. During the early stages, however, it may take a beginner about 80–90 seconds to perform one repetition. It is unnecessary to concern yourself with the amount of time required to perform breathing exercise. As you become more accustomed to doing it, the time required will decrease. It is necessary, however, to develop a sense of passing time and to learn how to count and adjust cadence before performing breathing exercise.

Manual for this breathing exercise: While the elapse of time is unimportant for the successful performance of breathing exercise, it is essential to bear in mind that inspiration must be coordinated with expiration. The regular respiration cycle should be within the range of from five to eight times per minute with an average minute ventilation of 6–10 liters. This type of respiration with the abdomen providing very little pressure, is similar to that described in Type 1. It is, therefore, thoracic respiration.

References: When this Type 2 breathing exercise is performed, the heart rate increases slightly, and the ratio of alpha waves, recorded by electroencephalogram, showed a decrease of 5.34 percent in the parietal region and a decrease of 3.66 percent in the occipital region. Among the nine basic breathing exercises, this Type 2

	Heart rate	Appearance rate of alpha wave	
		Parietal	Occipital
During exercise (A)	83.6	49.3	81.75
After exercise (B)	86.0	43.96	78.09
(A)−(B)	−2.4	+5.34	+3.66

Subject	Minute Respiration Cycle	Minute Ventilation (l)	Tidal Volume (l)	Minute Oxygen Consumption	Minute Carbon Dioxide Metabolism	Respiratory Quotient
A	6.7	7.96	1.35	0.261	0.282	1.112
B	6.0	5.60	0.925	0.151	0.188	1.245
C	8.0	12.40	1.55	0.347	0.414	1.196
Mean	6.9	8.65	1.275	0.253	0.295	1.166

breathing exercise ranks first in terms of changes in alpha wave ratio in the parietal region and fourth in terms of change in alpha wave ratio in the occipital region.

Things to be remembered: In order to perform breathing exercise properly, it is necessary to remember to keep your posture upright, to inhale and exhale only through the nose and to coordinate the time required for expiration and inspiration. Exercise time should be limited to between three and five minutes per repetition. You should make it a point to ensure that no repetition of your exercise exceeds this five minute limit. For the best results, this exercise should be performed regularly, three times every day—in the morning, afternoon and evening.

Type 3. Seven by seven breathing method

Keep your posture upright, and perform the breathing exercise described in Type 1 three times. Then, purse your lips and expel all air from the lungs through the mouth in one draught in an attempt to empty the lungs completely. Exhale, "foon." While exhaling, try to contract your belly and raise your diaphragm as high as possible. Hold your breath after exhaling. Then, keep your body relaxed and count "one, two, three." Slowly inhale through the nose, while counting "one, two, three, four, five, six, seven." Hei, hold your breath, while keeping your posture intact, and count "one, two." Then exhale slowly through the nose, while counting "one, two, three, four, five, six, seven." Then, hold your breath and count "one, two." Inhale slowly through the nose, while counting "one, two, three, four, five, six, seven." Hei hold your breath and count "one, two." Exhale slowly through the nose, while counting "one, two, three, four, five, six, seven."

Perform fourteen repetitions of this type of breathing exercise. It should take about three minutes. In the beginning, you may feel some strain in counting continuously to seven. If this is the case, adjust the amount of air inhaled so that you feel less strain. This exercise pattern is one of the easiest of the nine patterns to master. It is also convenient for people who are quite busy because it is suitable for performance while walking or strolling around. For example, start walking by stepping off with the left foot. Inhale through the nose, while walking, counting one, two, three, four, five, six, seven steps. Then, hold your breath for two steps. Finally, exhale through the nose, while walking, counting one, two, three, four, five, six, seven steps. It also is possible to perform this exercise on trains and buses every morning and evening because this type of exercise does not require any heavy spiritual concentration.

Manual for this breathing exercise: It is essential to the performance of this type of exercise that one not pay close attention to the passage of time. There is, however, an acute need to coordinate the time required for inspiration and required for expiration. An average respiration cycle for this pattern of exercise is between four and eight times per minute, and the ventilatory volume ranges from

	Heart rate	Appearance rate of alpha wave	
		Parietal	Occipital
During exercise (A)	83.8	49.43	78.87
After exercise (B)	90.0	44.72	82.32
(A)−(B)	−6.2	+4.71	−3.45

Subject	Minute Respiration Cycle	Minute Ventilation (l)	Tidal Volume (l)	Minute Oxygen Consumption	Minute Carbon Dioxide Metabolism	Respiratory Quotient
A	4.1	6.92	1.67	0.229	0.247	1.079
B	4.1	4.30	1.05	0.126	0.159	1.262
C	4.0	8.20	2.10	0.225	0.250	1.111
Mean	4.07	6.47	1.589	0.193	0.219	1.135

5 to 8 liters per minute. This pattern of exercise also creates rather strong pressure within the abdomen, when compared to those of Type 1 and Type 2. Among the nine patterns of respiration now under study, this pattern ranks sixth in terms of strengthening the abdominal region. It is permissible to say that this respiration method is located midway between thoracic and abdominal breathing.

References: The heart rate observed in subjects who have finished this pattern of breathing exercise is consistently higher than that registered while the same subjects were performing the exercise.

The ratio of alpha waves, recorded by electroencephalogram, showed a decrease of 4.71 percent in the parietal region and an increase of 3.45 percent in the occipital region. In each case, Type 3 breathing exercise ranks third among the nine basic breathing exercises.

Things to be remembered: Keep your posture upright, and breathe through your nose. Remember to coordinate the length of your inspiration with that of your expiration. It does not matter where this pattern of exercise is performed. You may do it whenever you like. However, it is important that you remember to practice at least twice every day—in the morning and evening—while sitting in a chiar.

Type 4. Treble breathing method

Keeping your posture upright, take a fresh breath, using the pattern explained in Type 1 three times. Pursing your lips, expel all air from the lungs in an attempt to empty them completely. Exhale, "foon." While exhaling, gradually contract your belly and raise your diaphragm as high as possible. After exhaling, hold your breath and count "one, two, three." Then, slowly inhale through the nose, while counting up to three, "one, two and three." Hei, hold your breath and count "one, two." Exhale slowly through the nose. while counting "one, two, three, four, five, six, seven, eight, nine." This is three times as many numbers as were counted during inspiration. (This means that it should take at least three times longer to exhale than it does to inhale.) After counting to nine, stop exhaling and hold your breath for a while. Then, inhale slowly through the nose, while counting up to four, "one, two, three, four." Hei, hold your breath for a while, while keeping your posture comfortable, and count "one, two." Exhale slowly through the nose, counting up to twelve, "one, two, three, four, five, six, seven, eight, nine, ten, eleven, twelve." Hei, hold your breath while counting, "one, two." Inhale slowly through the nose, while counting up to five, "one, two, three, four, five." Hei, hold your breath while counting, "one, two." Exhale slowly through the nose, counting up to fifteen, "one, two, three, four, five, six, seven, eight, nine, ten, eleven, twelve, thirteen, fourteen, fifteen." Hei, hold your breath while counting, "one, two." Then, inhale slowly through the nose, while counting up to six, "one, two, three, four, five, six." Hei, hold your breath while counting, "one, two." Exhale slowly through the nose, while counting up to eighteen, "one, two, three, four, five, six, seven, eight, nine, ten, eleven, twelve, thirteen, fourteen, fifteen, sixteen, seventeen, eighteen." Hei, hold your breath while counting, "one, two." Inhale slowly through the nose, while counting up to seven, "one, two, three, four, five, six, seven." Hei, hold your breath, while keeping your posture comfortable, and count, "one, two." Then, exhale slowly through the nose, while counting up to twenty-one, "one, two, three, four, five, six, seven, eight, nine, ten, eleven, twelve, thirteen, fourteen, fifteen, seventeen, eighteen, nineteen, twenty, twenty-one." Hei, hold your breath, keeping your posture natural. Inhale slowly through the nose, while counting up to seven again, "one, two, three, four, five, six, seven." Hei, hold your breath, while keeping your posture comfortable, and count, "one, two." Exhale slowly through the nose, while counting up to twenty-one, "one, two, three, four, five, six, seven, eight, nine, ten, eleven, twelve, thirteen, fourteen, fifteen, sixteen, seventeen, eighteen, nineteen, twenty, twenty-one." Hei, hold your breath, while keeping your posture natural, and count, "one, two." Inhale slowly through the nose, while counting up to six, "one, two, three, four, five, six." Hei, hold your breath, while keeping your posture natural, and count, "one, two." Exhale slowly through the nose, while counting up to eighteen, "one, two, three, four, five, six, seven, eight, nine, ten, eleven, twelve, thirteen, fourteen, fifteen, sixteen, seventeen, eighteen." Hei, hold your breath, while keeping your posture natural, and count, "one, two." Inhale slowly through the nose, while counting up to five, "one, two, three, four, five." Hei, hold your breath, while keeping your posture natural and count, "one, two." Exhale slowly through the nose, while counting up to fifteen, "one, two, three, four, five, six, seven, eight, nine, ten, eleven, twelve, thirteen, fourteen, fifteen." Hei, hold your breath, while keeping your posture comfortable, and count, "one, two." Inhale slowly through the nose, while counting up to four, "one, two, three, four." Hei, hold your breath and count, "one, two." Exhale slowly through the nose, while counting up to twelve, "one, two, three, four, five, six, seven, eight, nine, ten, eleven, twelve." Hei, hold your breath and count, "one, two." Inhale slowly through the nose, while counting up to three, "one, two, three." Hei, hold your breath and count, "one, two." Then, exhale slowly through the nose, while counting up to nine, "one, two, three, four, five, six, seven, eight, nine." Hei, this concludes the pattern.

In this exercise pattern, the inspiration time is increased by a count of from three, at the beginning, to a count of seven, and the time spent in expiration is increased proportionally from nine to twenty-one. After reaching the high point of seven counts for inspiration and twenty-one for expiration, the counts for each element of respiration are progressively decreased from twenty-one to nine for expiration and from seven to three for inspiration. It should take about three minutes and 30–50 seconds to complete a full repetition of this pattern of breathing exercise. You may find this exercise difficult at first, but once you have become accustomed to it, you should find it rather refreshing. Please remember, when performing this exercise, that all expiration must take place through the nose. Since this exercise is designed to require three times as much time for expiration as it does for inspiration, you must be ever conscious of always calculating the amount of air remaining in your lungs and must carefully control the volume of air exhaled. Otherwise, you may suffer strains in various parts of your body and may experience an unexpected setback in your performance of breathing exercise. If you find yourself faced with a problem when performing this pattern of breathing exercise, such as having no air left in your lungs before you have finished counting, you must stop the exercise and resume normal breathing. Then, after having rested for four or five minutes, you may attempt the exercise again.

Manual for this breathing exercise: In performing this exercise, you must focus your attention on expiration—expiration time must be three times as long as inspiration time. The average respiration cycle is between 2.5 and 4 times per minute and ventilatory volume ranges from 5.5 to 7.6 liters per minute. This respiration pattern is characterized by greater abdominal pressure than the other breathing patterns discussed to this point. Therefore, it could be said that this method is one step closer to abdominal respiration than those introduced above.

References: The heart rate observed in subjects who have finished this pattern

	Heart rate	Appearance rate of alpha wave	
		Parietal	Occipital
During exercise (A)	82.8	48.13	81.52
After exercise (B)	84.0	57.57	84.52
(A)−(B)	−1.2	−9.44	−3.00

Subject	Minute Respiration Cycle	Minute Ventilation (l)	Tidal Volume (l)	Minute Oxygen Consumption	Minute Carbon Dioxide Metabolism	Respiratory Quotient
A	3.23	6.49	1.92	0.227	0.205	0.893
B	3.55	4.00	1.13	0.164	0.118	0.719
C	3.00	7.50	2.50	0.236	0.225	0.952
Mean	3.26	5.99	1.85	0.209	0.182	0.854

of breathing exercise is consistently higher than that registered by the same subjects while performing the exercise. The ratio of alpha waves, recorded by electroencephalogram, showed an increase of 9.44 percent in the parietal region and an increase of 3.0 percent in the occipital region. Among the nine basic breathing patterns, this Type 4 pattern ranks second in terms of change in alpha wave ratio in the parietal region and ranks first in terms of change in the alpha wave ratio in the occipital region.

Things to be remembered: First, keep your posture upright and breathe through your nose during the exercise. Remember that, in this pattern, expiration should take three times as long as inspiration. You should avoid hard training, but two repetitions of the exercise should be done whenever it is performed. Take at least five-minutes of complete rest immediately after performing this pattern of exercise. During this rest period, breathe normally and refrain from smoking. Also avoid any immoderate exercise immediately after having performed this pattern of breathing exercise. (Do not take any physical exercise until at least ten minutes have passed.)

Type 5. Snuffle-snuffle type of breathing method

This pattern of exercise is very difficult to perform precisely. Therefore, only those who have mastered the four above described patterns of exercise are qualified to attempt this pattern.

The first step is to assume an upright posture and to perform three repetitions of the exercise described in Type 1. Next, purse your lips and expel all of the air from your lungs through your mouth in an attempt to empty your lungs completely. Then, try to raise your diaphragm as high as possible. After exhaling completely, hold your breath. Then, keeping your posture natural, count "one, two, three." Inhale through the nose, filling the lungs to their full capacity. (No particular instructions are given.) After inhaling fully, hold your breath and count, "one, two." Then exhale, through the nose, continuously in a series of short puffing actions, "snuffle, snuffle, snuffle." When no more air can be expelled through the nose, purse your lips and expel all remaining air through the mouth so that the lungs are completely empty.

Remember that your posture must remain upright at all times. Do not twist your body or you should experience a choking sensation. After expelling all air from the lungs, hold your breath and count, "one, two, three, four, five, six, seven, eight, nine, ten." After counting up to ten, inhale slowly through the nose. Be careful, however, not to draw mucus or saliva into the trachea. If you are confused or flustered, you may be seized by a fit of coughing. Therefore, inhale as slowly and as quiet as possible. Inhale to full capacity. Then, hold your breath and count, "one, two." Then, expel air from the lungs, gradually, in a series of short puffiing actions, "snuffle, snuffle, snuffle." When no more air can be expelled from the lungs by puffing through the nose, purse your lips and expel all remaining air through the mouth, "foon." Then, hold your breath and count up to fifteen. "one, two, three, four, five, six, seven, eight, nine, ten, eleven, twelve, thirteen, fourteen, fifteen." After counting, inhale through the nose. Having inhaled to the full capacity of the lungs, hold your breath and count, "one, two." Puff the air out through the nose, "snuffle, snuffle, snuffle." After puffing as much air as possible out through the nose, purse your lips and expel all remaining air through the mouth, "foon." Hei, hold your breath and count up to twenty, "one, two, three, four, five, six, seven, eight, nine, ten, eleven, twelve, thirteen, fourteen, fifteen, sixteen, seventeen, eighteen, nineteen, twenty." Having counted up to twenty, inhale through the nose slowly. After having inhaled to the full capacity of the lungs, hold your breath and count, "one, two." Then, expel air through the nose in a series of short puffing actions, "snuffle, snuffle, snuffle." After puffing as much air as possible out through the nose, purse your lips and expel all remaining air through the mouth, "foon." Hold your breath and count up to twenty-five, "one, two, three, four, five, six, seven, eight, nine, ten, eleven, twelve, thirteen, fourteen, fifteen, sixteen, seventeen, eighteen, nineteen, twenty, twenty-one, twenty-two, twenty-three, twenty-four, twenty-five." After counting, inhale through the nose slowly. Having inhaled to the full capacity of the lungs, hold your breath and count, "one, two." Then, expel air through the nose in puffing actions, "snuffle, snuffle, snuffle." After exhaling all air from the nose, then, purse your lips and expel the air from the mouth this time, "foon." Then, hold your breath and count up to thirty, "one, two, three, four, five, six, seven, eight, nine, ten, eleven, twelve, thirteen, fourteen, fifteen, sixteen, seventeen, eighteen, nineteen, twenty, twenty-one, twenty-two, twenty-three, twenty-four, twenty-five, twenty-six, twenty-seven, twenty-eight, twenty-nine, thirty." After counting, inhale through the nose. After having counted up to a high of thirty during the phase when you are holding your breath, perform the exercise in reverse, decreasing the count from thirty to twenty-five to twenty to fifteen and, finally, to ten.

It should take some three minutes and thirty seconds to perform a full repetition of this exercise pattern. This is a very difficult exercise, and those performing it sometimes experience a choking sensation. Therefore, do not force yourself to perform this practice. Once you become accustomed to it, however, you will feel refreshed and will enjoy a renewed vitality each time that you perform the exercise. While exhaling air through the nose in a series of puffs, you must contract your abdominal region gradually. And when expelling air through the mouth, try to contract your abdomen further. To stop breathing, constrict the throat.

If you relax your abdomen while holding your breath, you will experience a sensation of the throat being drawn down into the lungs. In order to avoid such a distressing sensation, you must carefully relax your body. When drawing air into the lungs through the nose, do not inhale quickly, even if you feel as though you are choking. It is important to inhale quietly and calmly as if you were tasting the air.

Manual for this breathing exercise: You must concentrate your attention on holding your breath after expiration. Fix your eyes on a point on the floor, and do not think about anything. If you have some physical defect in your body, then concentrate your attention on that. You must imagine that while you are holding your breath, the physical deficiency is being removed by some powerful sucking force.

Inhale naturally, without paying any particular attention to doing so, but do draw the air into the lungs in separate motions, repeatedly, in order to regulate your respiration. Do not forget that the inspiration has to be done in one deep draught.

The average respiratory cycle of this exercise is between 1.5 and 3 times per minute. and ventilatory volume is around 3 to 5 liters per minute, As for abdominal pressure in this pattern of breathing exercise, it is regarded as being rather strong compared with abdominal pressures in the remainder of the nine basic breathing exercises. But the total pressure imposed on the abdominal region during this fifth exercise pattern is near zero, because negative pressure is imposed on the region while holding the breath, and this negative pressure offsets the positive pressure imposed on the abdominal parts while exhaling and inhaling actions are performed.

References: The heart rate observed in subjects who have finished this pattern

	Heart rate	Appearance rate of alpha wave	
		Parietal	Occipital
During exercise (A)	81.7	40.62	67.54
After exercise (B)	84.0	47.05	86.32
(A)−(B)	−2.3	−6.43	−18.78

Subject	Minute Respiration Cycle	Minute Ventilation (l)	Tidal Volume (l)	Minute Oxygen Consumption	Minute Carbon Dioxide Metabolism	Respiratory Quotient
A	1.95	4.36	2.26	0.198	0.177	0.851
B	3.15	3.60	1.14	0.121	0.116	0.958
C	2.00	3.50	1.75	0.175	0.155	0.890
Mean	2.37	3.82	1.72	0.165	0.149	0.899

of breathing exercise is slight higher than that registered by the same subjects while performing the exercise.

The alpha wave rate, recorded by electroencephalogram, showed an increase of 6.43 percent in the parietal region and 18.78 percent in the occipital region when compared with those rates recorded during the exercise.

Among the nine basic breathing practice patterns, this Type 5 pattern ranks eighth in terms of change in the alpha wave rate in the parietal region and second in terms of change in the occipital region. However, the margin of fluctuation between the alpha waves rates observed during the exercise and those observed after is greater than the margin observed in any of the other nine basic exercises.

Things to be remembered: Do not force yourself to perform this exercise, but try to perform at least one repetition of this pattern per day. It is desirable to temper the frequency of the exercise to the physical conditions of the exerciser. Do not perform this Type 5 exercise in conjunction with the Type 4 exercise. Rest quietly for about ten minutes after this exercise and also refrain from smoking for about fifteen minutes.

Type 6. Broken wind breathing method

This pattern of exercise is even more difficult than the Type 5 pattern. There-fore, only those who have completely mastered the patterns of exercise described in Types 1 through 5 are qualified to attempt this pattern exercise. Those suffering from hypertension and heart disease are strictly prohibited from performing this Type 6 exercise. If they were to attempt this exercise, they might encounter an unexpected setback or an accident.

Keep your posture upright. Perform three repetitions of the deep breathing exercise described in Type 1. Then pursuing your lips, expel all air from the lungs through the mouth in an attempt to empty the lungs completely, "foon." Re-member to gradually raise the diaphragm as high as possible, while contracting the abdominal region. Having exhaled, hold your breath. Then, relax your body and count "one, two." Inhale through the nose slowly, while counting up to fourteen, "one, two, three, four, five, six, seven, eight, nine, ten, eleven, twelve, thirteen, fourteen." Hei, hold your breath while counting up to twenty, "one, two, three, four, five, six, seven, eight, nine, ten, eleven, twelve, thirteen, fourteen, fifteen, sixteen, seventeen, eighteen, nineteen, twenty." Exhale through the nose slowly, forcing all air out of the lungs vigorously. After exhaling, reorder your respiration by breathing normally three times. Now, inhale through the nose slowly while counting up to fourteen, "one, two, three, four, five, six, seven, eight, nine, ten, eleven, twelve, thirteen, fourteen." Hei, hold your breath while counting up to twenty-five, "one, two, three, four, five, six, seven, eight, nine, ten, eleven, twelve, thirteen, fourteen, fifteen, sixteen, seventeen, eighteen, nineteen, twenty, twenty-one, twenty-two, twenty-three, twenty-four, twenty-five." Exhale through the nose slowly, but once again, force all air through the nose vigorously, in an attempt to empty the lungs completely. Having exhaled all air from the lungs, take breath naturally four times, in an attempt to regulate your respiration. Then, inhale through the nose slowly while counting up to fourteen, "one, two, three, four, five, six, seven, eight, nine, ten, eleven, twelve, thirteen, fourteen." Hei, hold your breath while counting up to thirty, "one, two, three, four, five, six, seven, eight, nine, ten, eleven, twelve, thirteen, fourteen, fifteen, sixteen, seventeen, eighteen, nineteen, twenty, twenty-one, twenty-two, twenty-three, twenty-four twenty-five, twenty-six, twenty-seven, twenty-eight, twenty-nine, thirty." Exhale through the nose slowly but forcefully in an attempt to expel all remaining air from the lungs. Then breathe naturally five times, in order to regulate your breathing. After counting up to thirty, reverse the progression, decreasing the count from thirty to twenty-five and finally, to twenty. This means that the length of time the breath is held will be shortened gradually (in this case, holding the breath creates positive pressure).

It should take about five minutes to perform one repetition of this exercise. Do not force yourself to do this exercise, as it can result in discomfort, particularly in that phase wherein you are required to hold your breath for a count of thirty before relaxing your body. At the beginning of this exercise, you may experience some difficulty and fatigue. They can be overcome, however. Therefore, strive hard during this difficult early period. These difficulties are actually an essential element of the exercise itself.

Manual for this breathing exercise: While holding your breath, concentrate your attention by staring at a point on the floor. If you have defects in your body, then concentrate your attention on that deficiency. Imagine that the physical defect is being pushed out of your body by some powerful force while you are holding your breath, and that you eagerly wish this fantasy to be realized.

The average respiration cycle is between 4.5–8 times per minute and ventilatory volume is about 4.5 to 7 liters per minute. The abdominal pressure associated with this exercise is higher than that of any of the nine basic breathing exercises. While the breath is held, huge positive pressure is placed on the abdominal region and sometimes, in addition, valsalva breath holding occurs.

References: The heart rate observed in subjects who have finished this pattern of breathing exercise is markedly less than that registered by the same subjects while performing the exercise. The alpha wave ratio, recorded by electroencephalogram, showed a marked decrease of 9.86 percent in the parietal region and a drop of 18.98 percent in the occipital region when compared with those ratios recorded during the exercise.

Among the nine basic breathing exercises, this Type 6 pattern ranks sixth in terms of change in the alpha wave ratio in the parietal region and eighth in terms of change in the occipital region.

Things to be remembered: Those suffering from heart defects or hypertension

	Heart rate	Appearance rate of alpha wave	
		Parietal	Occipital
During exercise (A)	87.4	39.15	71.18
After exercise (B)	80.0	29.29	52.20
(A)−(B)	+7.4	+9.86	+18.98

Subject	Minute Respiration Cycle	Minute Ventilation (l)	Tidal Volume (l)	Minute Oxygen Consumption	Minute Carbon Dioxide Metabolism	Respiratory Quotient
A	5.05	5.19	1.048	0.215	0.201	0.938
B	5.65	5.75	1.02	0.127	0.120	0.945
C	6.00	6.50	1.08	0.221	0.201	0.911
Mean	5.57	5.81	1.049	0.187	0.174	0.931

or hemorrhoids are strictly prohibited from undergoing this exercise.

All the other respiration exercises should be performed separately from this pattern of exercise. This is to avoid unexpected adverse affects which may result from the accelerating effects of this exercise. After performing the exercise, inhale and exhale sufficiently to fully relax the muscles used for breathing.

Type 7. Windup breathing method

In this exercise, in the same manner as a baseball pitcher preparing to throw, the exerciser winds his arm continuously through six revolutions while inhaling through the nose (Figs. 36 through 38). Then wind the arm in reverse through another six revolutions, while exhaling through the nose. After exhaling all air through the nose, quickly clench the fist and raise it over the head while inhaling through the nose (Fig. 39). Then, bend the upper body forward and put the knuckles down on the floor (Figs. 40 and 41). During this motion, hold your breath. Having touched the floor, gradually raise the upper body and lift the arm above the head. Rotating the arm backward, place it alongside the body while smoothly exhaling through the nose.

Then, change arms and repeat the same sequence of actions. The times to be spent for each of these actions are as follows:
1) six seconds for inspiration
2) six seconds for expiration
3) two seconds for inspiration
4) four seconds for holding the breath
5) eight seconds for expiration
6) four seconds for holding the breath

It should take about one minute for one repetition of this exercise with each arm.

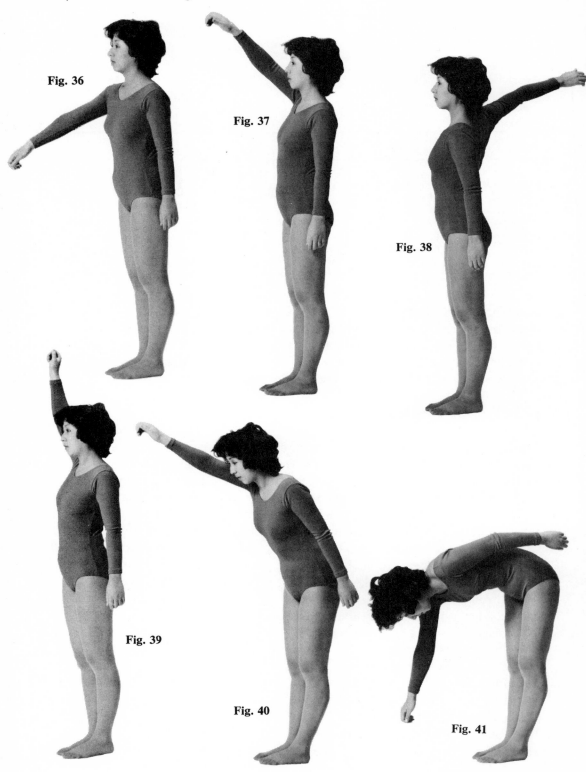

Fig. 36

Fig. 37

Fig. 38

Fig. 39

Fig. 40

Fig. 41

This pattern of exercise is rather confusing. Therefore, it will take some time to become accustomed to it. However, after learning the ropes of the exercise, you should have no difficulty in performing it. The key is to coordinate the respiration cycle with the movements of the arms and waist. Once you have accomplished this, comfortable and pleasant breathing exercise will be within your grasp.

Manual for this breathing exercise: Remember that the smooth flow of regular breathing must be coordinated with the movements of the arms and waist. This derived from the time-honored art of Japanese dance. The average respiration cycle is about 4 times per minute and ventilatory volume is about 10 liters per minute. This exercise pattern is believed to result in greater abdominal pressures than most of the other eight basic breathing exercises.

References: The heart rate observed in subjects who have finished this pattern of breathing exercise is markedly less than that registered by the same subjects when performing the exercise. The alpha wave ratio recorded by electroencephalogram after the exercise showed a considerable decrease of 6.56 percent in the parietal region and a considerable increase of 6.03 percent in the occipital region when compared with those ratios recorded during the exercise.

Among the nine basic breathing exercises, this pattern ranks seventh in terms of change in the alpha wave ratio in the parietal region and ninth in the terms of change in the occipital region.

	Heart rare	Appearance rate of alpha wave	
		Parietal	Occipital
During exercise (A)	79.6	42.67	68.09
After exercise (B)	74.0	36.11	74.12
(A)−(B)	+5.6	+6.56	−6.03

Subject	Minute Respiration Cycle	Minute Ventilation (l)	Tidal Volume (l)	Minute Oxygen Consumption	Minute Carbon Dioxide Metabolism	Respiratory Quotient
A	3.07	7.46	2.42	0.429	0.386	0.900
B	6.20	6.50	1.05	0.300	0.240	0.840
C	4.00	10.00	2.50	0.450	0.420	0.933
Mean	4.42	7.98	1.99	0.393	0.349	0.887

Things to be remembered: Remember not to turn your arms in wrong direction. Also, remember to inhale and exhale through the nose. Try to extend, gradually and proportionally, as in previously described patterns, the time spent inhaling, exhaling and holding your breath. Top priority must be given to coordinating the respiration cycle with the movements of the arms and waist.

If the body is stiff, do not try this exercise without first warming-up properly. Considerable time should be spent bending and stretching the waist in order to be able to touch the fist to the floor without bending the knees. Once you can do this, you may perform this pattern of exercise.

Do not tighten the arm while winding it up. Instead, relax it as smoothly as possible.

Type 8. Pit and corn breathing method

The most important characteristic of this pattern of breathing exercise is that it can be performed whenever and wherever the execiser wishes, even while walking or standing. There is no particular way to stand or walk when performing this exercise. Just remember to keep the weight on the ball or thenar of the foot. The secret to successful performance of this exercise is to keep your toes turned slightly inward while standing or walking.

First, maintain an upright posture. Next, perform three repetitions of the breathing exercise described in Type 1. Then, pursing your lips, expel all of the air from your lungs, "foon." Gradually contract the abdomen, while exhaling, and attempt to raise the diaphragm. Having exhaled, hold your breath and relax your body, while counting up to three, "one, two, three." Raise both arms forward to shoulder level, while slowly inhaling through the nose. Next, extend your arm, wrists, and hands in a straight line at shoulder height. Turn your palms downward and extend your fingers (Fig. 42). Then, exhaling through the nose slowly, relax your hands and fingers and permit your hands to droop downward (Fig. 43). Slowly inhale through the nose, while forcefully extending your arms, wrists and fingers in a straight line. Slowly exhale, while relaxing your arms, wrists and fingers and permitting your hands to droop downward. Repeat this pattern of exercise three times. While inhaling through the nose for fourth time, rotate your arms backward while keeping them extended horizontally. Rotate your arms to the point where they can go no further. Then, forcefully extend your arms, wrists and fingers in a straight line (Fig. 44). At this point, inspiration should be completed. Next, exhale through the nose while relaxing your arms, wrists and fingers (Fig. 45). Slowly inhale through the nose, while forcefully extending your arms, wrists, and fingers. While slowly exhaling through the nose, relax your arms, wrists and fingers and permit your hands to hang downward. Repeat this exercise three times. Lower your arms slowly and place them along side of your body, while exhaling slowly through the nose for the seventh time. This exercise is complete once you have repeated three repetitions of the described exercise.

Remember that this pattern of exercise must be performed with gracefulness. You should resemble a crane flying across the sky with its big wings fully extended.

Fig. 42

Fig. 43

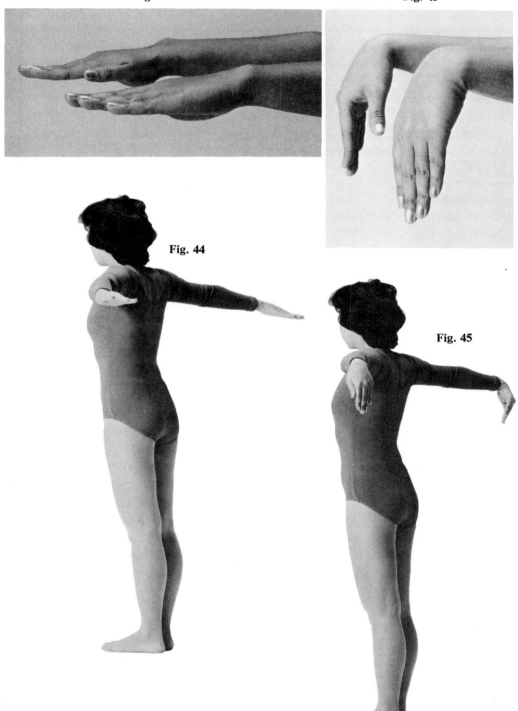

Fig. 44

Fig. 45

Manual for this breathing exercise: Remember to coordinate the motion of your arms, wrists and fingers with the rhythm of your breathing. The key to this exercise lies in leisurely actions. Therefore, do not rush while performing this pattern of exercise. The average respiration cycle for this exercise is between five and eight times per minute, and ventilatory volume is about 9.0 to 14 liters per minute. This pattern of exercise generates the least abdominal pressure of any of the nine basic breathing exercise patterns.

References: The heart rate observed in subjects who have finished this exercise does not differ from that registered by the same subject while performing the exercise. However, alpha wave ratios, recorded after the exercise showed substantial increases, 11.06 percent in the parietal region and 7.37 percent in the occipital region, over those rates recorded during the exercise. Among the nine basic breathing patterns, this ranks fifth in terms of change in alpha wave ratio in the parietal region and ranks sixth in terms of change in the occipital region.

	Heart rate	Appearance rate of alpha wave	
		Parietal	Occipital
During exercise (A)	76.4	45.49	73.94
After exercise (B)	78.0	56.55	81.31
(A)−(B)	−1.6	−11.06	−7.37

Subject	Minute Respiration Cycle	Minute Ventilation (l)	Tidal Volume (l)	Minute Oxygen Consumption	Minute Carbon Dioxide Metabolism	Respiratory Quotient
A	4.87	9.77	2.01	0.331	0.373	1.127
B	8.65	8.90	1.03	0.285	0.293	1.028
C	3.50	6.00	1.71	0.234	0.243	1.038
Mean	5.67	8.22	1.58	0.283	0.303	1.071

Things to be remembered: Establish an order for the performance of this exercise, so that you do not become flustered. Remember to perform this pattern of exercise as slowly and as smoothly as possible. Allow for some latitude of action by relaxing the movements of the knees and waist. Distinguish between those actions while must be performed deliberately and those which may be performed leisurely.

Type 9. High-tension breathing method

This breathing exercise may be performed while sitting in a chair. Therefore, it may be performed whenever and wherever you wish. Maintain an erect posture.

Next, perform three repetitions of the deep breathing exercise described in Type 1. Then, while pursing your lips, exhale all air from the lungs, "foon." While expelling air, contract your abdomen gradually and attempt to raise your diaphragm. After exhaling, hold your breath. Having held your breath, relax your body while counting to three, "one, two, three." While sitting on a chair, grasp the seat of the chair firmly with both hands and pull up with all of your strength as if in an attempt of lift the chair (Fig. 46). Further contract your arms, abdomen and other muscles still as in an attempt to lift the seat on which you are sitting, and inhale through the nose. Keeping your body in a highly tense condition, hold your breath. (The length of the time breathing is held should be varied for each exerciser, depending on the condition of his health.) Exhale through the nose slowly, while relaxing your body and releasing your grip on the chair. Relax your whole body completely after exhaling through the nose. There should be no tension in any part of your body at this time. Complete the exercise by performing three repetitions of the pattern described above. Remember to adjust the length of expiration, inspiration and the period for which the breath is held in accordance with the condition of your health and your breathing rhythm.

Fig. 46   **Fig. 47**

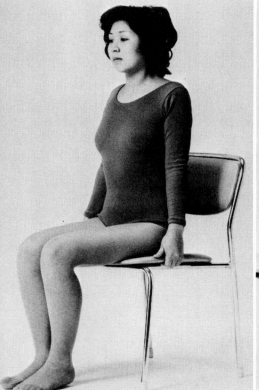
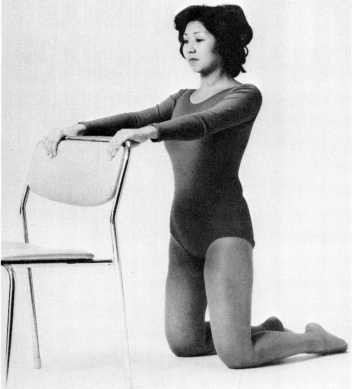

Variations of this exercise may be performed while standing straight or lying on the floor. Furthermore, it even can be performed while kneeling, provided that you keep your upper body erect and support yourself by holding onto the back of a chair (Fig. 47).

A simple exercise is to make your body tense while inhaling, to hold your breath, and, finally, to relax while exhaling through the nose. This exercise may be performed while riding in a train, a bus, a car, or even an aircraft. For instance, while hanging from a strap in the commuter train or bus, increase the tension in your body while inhaling, hold your breath and then, relax while exhaling. When driving your own car, you can perform this exercise while you are stopped or waiting for a green light. Hold the wheel firmly in your hands and press down on the brake pedal with your foot. Then, inhale, hold your breath for a moment while tense, and then relax while exhaling. Remember, however, not to try this while actually driving your car.

Manual for this breathing exercise: Those people suffering from hypertension, heart ailment, and hemorrhoids are not permitted to perform this exercise. Even other people are urged to exercise caution. Do not strain too forcefully from the beginning and, after straining, relax your body for a while. This is absolutely necessary in order to maintain balance between inspiration and expiration. Once you have learned how to coordinate your respiration, continue your exercise at a level appropriate for yourself.

The average respiration cycle for this pattern of exercise is between two and four times per minute and ventilatory volume ranges between 3.5 and 5.0 liters per minute. Of the nine basic patterns, this breathing exercise imposes the highest pressure on the abdominal region.

References: It is difficult to accurately measure heart rate during this exercise, because the electrocardiograph does not operate normally due to the influence of the electricity caused by muscular stimulation.

The alpha wave ratio was found to have increases slightly, 0.8 percent in the parietal region after exercise, when compared with the ratio recorded during the exercise. However a significant increase of 29.84 percent was observed in the occipital region after exercise when compared with the ratio registered in that area during the exercise.

	Heart rate	Appearance rate of alpha wave	
		Parietal	Occipital
During exercise (A)	unavailable	33.68	49.25
After exercise (B)	70.0	34.48	79.09
(A)−(B)		−0.8	−29.84

Subject	Minute Respiration Cycle	Minute Ventilation (l)	Tidal Volume (l)	Minute Oxygen Consumption	Minute Carbon Dioxide Metabolism	Respiratory Quotient
A	2.54	4.55	1.79	0.227	0.197	0.868
B	6.65	7.00	1.05	0.293	0.273	0.932
C	1.80	3.24	1.80	0.293	0.234	0.799
Mean	3.66	4.93	1.55	0.271	0.235	0.867

Among the nine basic breathing exercises, this pattern ranks last in terms of change in the alpha wave ratio in the parietal region and first in terms of change in the occipital region. This proves that this pattern of exercise is superior to the other breathing exercises.

Things to be remembered: Remember that balance must be maintained between high inspiration and relaxed expiration.
Beginners commonly make the following mistakes:

1. They become tired quickly because they assume an incorrect posture.
2. They inhale through the nose too quickly and, as a result, they suffer from coughing fits and shortness of breath.
3. They may become exasperated or suffer headaches if breathing rhythms are changed and the balance between the respiration cycle and the alternate straining and relaxing is lost. In extreme cases, they may become nauseated or begin to vomit.
4. They may experience an icy sensation in the tips of the fingers and the forehead while performing the exercises described in Types 5 and 6. (Do not be concerned, continue to exercise steadily, but at a slightly slower pace depending on the condition of your health.)
5. Those who are suffering from hypertension, heart ailments and other diseases of this type are strictly prohibited from performing the exercises described in Types 5 and 6.
6. It is difficult to see the effects of these breathing exercises after performing them for only a couple of days. Therefore, bear in mind that it is necessary to be patient and steadfast and to adhere to a specific program worked out in accordance with the authorized instructions.

Six Steps in Authentic Oriental Breathing Therapy

In breathing therapy in the Orient, various breathing methods are employed to keep the body in good health by enhancing the function of each body organ, adjusting abnormalities within the body and at the same time eradicating causes of diseases. Since olden times, numerous studies have been made in an effort to find an ideal method of respiration. In Japan and China, in particular, active research on breathing methods has recently been performed not only by physicians, psychologists and physical education specialists but also by the general public.

As a result, six standard methods of respiration have been established. Acupuncture, shiatsu, *amma* and moxibustion, all of which are related to these breathing methods which form a core of Oriental medicine. In order, these six steps consist of (1) respiration via the abdomen, (2) circulating air through the upper half of the body, (3) circulating air throughout the body, (4) slow abdominal type respiration, (5) strengthened deep breathing and (6) respiration for coordinating mind and body.

The above respiration methods are listed in order of difficulty in exercise. Since advancing to a higher step skipping intermediate steps could result in unexpected accidents, it is essential to master each step with the utmost care.

Step 1 (Learning the method of lengthen the respiratory cycle)

The first step begins by voluntarily controlling normal breathing by extending the respiration period. For this purpose, "Form of Three Circles" in the erect position should be taken (see p. 40).
   —First, exhale slowly from the mouth. (Breathe out while puckering up your mouth.) This should be done smoothly without exertion.
   —During expiration, bring the upper teeth into light contact with the lower teeth.
   —When the expiration cycle is complete, slowly breathe in through the nose. The mouth should be closed and upper and lower teeth should remain in light contact. Breathe in while narrowing the nasal cavity slightly. This will create a partial restriction of the incoming air and thus increase the amount of time required for breathing in a given amount of air.
In this way, the respiration cycle period is gradually lengthened. The air of the Step 1 is to make respiration last long in a natural way, not little by little as mentioned in Type 2 of "Nine Basic Methods for Breathing Exercise" in which exercise of long respiration is made while counting the number of inspirations and expirations.

During the inspiration period, the friction of the air on the side and rear walls of the nasal cavity generates a pleasurable sensation in the brain. In addition, total concentration on the breathing sound felt through the nasal cavity has a soothing effect of tranquilizing the nerves. The exercise in Step 1 should be determined in accordance with the physical condition of each individual, but a general rule-of-thumb guide is three to four minutes per exercise. Prior to exercising Step 1, relieve tension mentally and physically by progressively relaxing shoulders and arms. This breathing exercise should also be done slowly and deliberately. As beginners are often unstable in their posture as well as their standing attitude of the "Form of Three Circles," it is necessary to fully practice and master

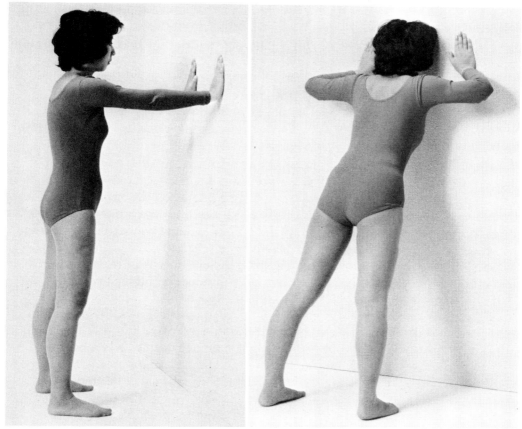

Fig. 48   **Fig. 49**

the proper stance. But, following method is also recommendable for them.

First, arrange both feet in line and stand 60 to 80 centimeters away from a wall, and facing a pole, a tree or a partner. Extend both arms toward the facing object and touch it (or her) with the palms of your hands (Fig. 48). (In this case, the body is bent forward slightly.)

—While breathing out, bend both arms and, by bending the upper half of the body forward, touch the facing object with the forehead (Fig. 49). This posture is kept until expiration is complete. In other words, the body is in an upright standing position at the initial stage of expiration, bends forward during expiration and ends the expiration cycle with the forehead touching the facing object.

—At the final stage of respiration, the breath is held for a while prior to the next process of inspiration.

—Inhale while gradually raising the body from the bent position of the expiration period.

—At the time of the maximum inspiration, the body is upright with both arms straight out.

—The breath is held during the transition period from the maximum inspiration to expiration.

When this method is thoroughly mastered, the beginner can advance to the original "Form of Three Circles" in the erect position.

If you have just recovered from an illness or if you are not feeling well, you must not carry the exercise too far. This exercise can be done by sitting on a chair or lying on the bed.

The major aim of Step 1 is to help, in a natural way, to slow down the rapid and erratic respiration (about 18 respirations per minute) of those who are not yet familiar with breathing control methods or those who have neglected basic training in respiration. Step 1 can be said to be a step in which the rudiments of "Junki" (correct and soft respiration) and "Yōki" (ample and strong respiration overflowing the body) are mastered. Step 1 is designed to strengthen the ventilation function of the lungs; promote the development of cells of the human body; and establish the foundation for further and additional breathing exercises.

If a person uses only thoracic respiration, he can be said to rely on a very wrong method of respiration. This type of respiration is achieved by moving the chest, which eventually causes the shoulders to move up and down. The reason why apical breathing is bad for health is that pulmonary apicitis can be caused by cool outside air inhaled into the apex of the lungs. Also, breathing by the use of shoulders take place mostly in such situations when we are excited, crying, tired, or ill.

Abdominal respiration is a method of respiration by which the abdomen is pushed out with inspiration and wide respiration surface is obtained. During this type of respiration, as the diaphragm is lowered, the abdomen is pushed out, and the chest capacity is expanded downward. This means that respiration is accomplished by the base of the lungs where the tissues are the strongest of all lung tissues. During the expiration, abdominal muscles contract allowing the abdomen to lower. As the diaphragm is pushed up, the lungs are pressurized through the action of the diaphragm to discharge contaminated air remaining in the corners of the lungs. Furthermore, the abdominal respiration method improves the circulation of blood throughout the circulatory system. Although arterial blood pushed out by the heart has a strong force, the heart itself does not draw in venous blood. Venous blood is returned from the abdomen to the heart by the contraction of elastic abdominal blood vessels and the diaphragm. Therefore, when the functions of the abdominal muscles and diaphragm are insufficient, venous blood is not circulated and remains in the abdomen. Hence, the importance of the abdominal respiration exercise.

Blood accounts for one-thirteenth of the weight of the human body (approximately 4 to 5 liters) and is circulated through the entire body. There are many people who suffer from illnesses because blood circulation is poor with perhaps a part of the entire blood supply becoming stagnant somewhere in their system.

Such people look pale, have cold limbs, get tired easily and suffer from stomach-aches and stiffness in their shoulders. Uncirculated blood stagnant in the abdominal region could be the cause. If the abdominal region relaxes, it follows that about two-thirds of the entire blood supply could stagnate there. In such a case, venous blood remains and congests in the stomach and the intestines, further impairing the blood circulation. To prevent this congestion of blood, it is necessary to concentrate on strengthening the abdominal region. With an increase in pressure in the abdominal region, venous blood is returned to the heart, normalizing blood circulation and resulting in energy returning to the whole body.

The abdominal region called "the abdominal heart" has an important nervous system consisting of the vagus nerve, the splanchnic nerve and other sympathetic nerves which have a direct connection with the sustenance of life. This area also contains a venous valve which meters the amount of blood circulating to and from the legs.

In addition, the walls of the stomach and intestines have their own plexuses which, when subjected to mechanical stimuli through abdominal respiration and pressure, function to enhance or suppress excitement, contract or expand vessels of the stomach and intestines and increase the secretion of gastrointestinal juices. These plexuses, when stimulated properly, also adjust the functions of the lungs and the heart by reflex action and they can affect vasomotoricity throughout the whole body for the improvement of blood circulation. By conducting a correct abdominal respiration straining the diaphragm, it becomes possible to shape a large-minded character.

When we are seized with fear, we bend forward and then shrink back. When the body bends forward suddenly, the diaphragm is raised and exerts pressure on the chest. Since most people inhale in such a case, even stronger pressure is applied to the chest and accordingly to the heart, which reacts by beating harder than usual. The diaphragm is a typical muscle which is related to the breathing exercise. When the diaphragm lowers, the thorax is expanded, while the abdominal cavity becomes narrower in inverse proportion to the expansion of the thorax. Thus, the stomach, intestines and other internal organs are pushed out in the forward lower direction. When the diaphragm is raised, the thorax is narrowed and the lungs are contracted. As a result, the stomach, intestines and other internal organs in the abdominal cavity come into the inside and the abdominal wall recedes. This motion is called a "diaphragm motion through respiration."

Step 2 (To draw in the abdomen during expiration and push it out during inspiration)

Use the "Form of Three Circles" in the erect position.
  —First exhale slowly through the mouth and then exercise Step 2.
  —While exhaling, bring the upper and lower teeth into light contact with each other.

Fig. 50

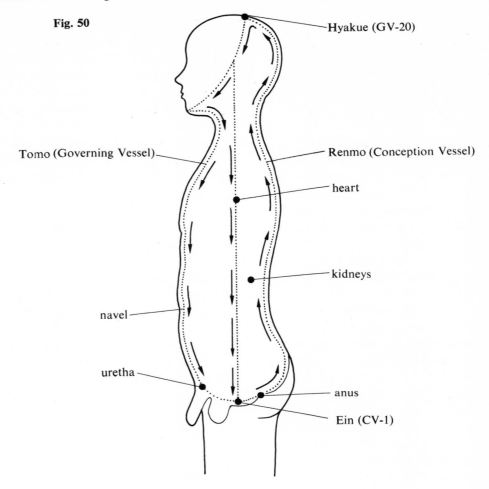

Hyakue (GV-20)

Tomo (Governing Vessel)

Renmo (Conception Vessel)

heart

kidneys

navel

uretha

anus

Ein (CV-1)

—After exhaling completely, inhale slowly through the nose. In this case, close the mouth, bring the upper and lower teeth into contact with each other and slightly narrow the nasal cavity.

This method of inspiration and expiration is the same as in Step 1. In case of expiration, however, contrary to Step 1, the abodiminal region is expanded while exhaling.

—After exhaling completely, inhale slowly through the nose.

In this case, the abdomiminal region is contracted slowly. (This is also contrary to Step 1.) While inhaling, try to scratch the ground with your toes and depress the upper jaw by means of the tip of the tongue. The upper jaw is the end of *Tomo* (governing vessel), while the end of the tongue is the end of the *Renmo* (conception vessel). Therefore, touching the upper jaw with the end of the tongue means that the conception vessel and the governing vessel are put together.

The fundamental difference between Oriental medicine and Western medicine should be noted, regarding the way of thinking, the logic in thinking and the approaches to diseases and patients. To be more specific, Western medicine places emphasis on the cure of a disease, while Oriental medicine emphasizes the cure of the patient. In the concept of curing a disease, a patient is left out of consideration, but in the concept of curing a patient, both mind and body of the patient are taken into consideration. In the case of Western medicine, treatment is impossible unless the disease of the patient is known. In other words, each disease is given a specific name with its remedy clearly defined. On the other hand, if the name of the disease is unknown, nothing can be done. Moreover, even a remedy for a certain disease cannot be recognized as such unless proven in actual cases as effective against identified causes of the disease.

On the other hand, Oriental medicine attaches importance not to how such and such a disease can be cured, but what medicine should be administered to a patient in order to relieve him of his pain. This way of thinking is one of the Oriental concepts entertained about diseases.

To be sure, the human body is made up of material, but material itself is controlled by "Ki" or energy. Diseases arise when this "Ki," flowing through the human body is diminishing or weakening, thus slowing down the functions of the human body. Essentially, the human body, overflowing with "Ki," is so designed as to live a healthy life and any bacillus or virus which invade the human body is no threat at all and easily discharged. Therefore, when we have fallen ill, it is necessary to fully replenish our bodies with "Ki" so as to make up for reduced or weakened "Ki" within it. To put it another way, "Ki" is, as previously mentioned, "unknown energy of life."

In the exercise of Step 2, extend both arms outward during expiration and fold them inside during inspiration. Distribute the force in outward extension and inward folding of the arms at the rate of three and seven, respectively. Once skill has been acquired in the above exercise, however, the exercise of expiration and inspiration should be made by not actual but imaginary motions of the arms. In other words, this breathing method is one which should be carried out only by imaging such arms motions.

The major advantages of the Step 2 exercise are a further development of the strengh of "Yōki" referred to in Step 1 and the enhancement of its medical effect. In general, repeated exercise of Step 2 for three months has the effect of gradually improving the reflex action sensitive to the central nerves, correcting the central nervous system of the brain and the spinal cord and curing chronic diseases of all kinds. This method also contributes toward gradually building up a sound and healthy body free from illness. Those who have completed three months' exercises may proceed to Step 3.

Those who are exercising Step 2 but are having difficulty with it are invited to try the following:

When inhaling, expand the abdominal region voluntarily and when exhaling, contract it also voluntarily with your waist pulled up and the anus tightened.

The aim in this exercise is to increase tension and relaxation of the abdominal region for acceleration of the internal circulation of "Kisoku," stimulate each nervous system and organ and strengthen the reflex action.

In Step 1, the abdominal region has been contracted at expiration and expanded at inspiration. In this case, the diaphragm expands only about 5 centimeters, which makes it impossible to apply a strong abdominal pressure to the abdominal region. However, by following the method of Step 2, it is possible to strengthen the function of the diaphragm to an extent that expands it by 13–15 centimeters. This is sufficient to apply a strong abdominal pressure to the abdominal region.

In this way, the breathing exercise in Step 2 is a thin, deep and long one in which the abdominal wall muscles are moved contrary to the method described for Step 1 and the area of motion of the diaphragm is expanded. Strengthening the function of the diaphragm contributes to increased ventilation volume by the lungs and increased pressure of the abdominal cavity. Peristalsis of the stomach and intestines promotes circulation and exchange of arterial and venous blood through capillary vessels. At the same time, it serves to pull up the anus and colon muscles for further strengthening of the abdominal cavity.

Therefore, blood circulation is enhanced for better metabolism by providing a rhythmic and comfortable stimulus and massage to each organ inside the abdominal cavity. This is carried out by the well-coordinated motion of the expansion and contraction of the abdominal muscles and wall and the up and down motion of the diaphragm. An increased appetite and better digestion are additional benefits which give the human body the strength to cure disease and keep the body in good health.

Step 3 (To master even thinner and longer respiration than in Step 2)

This Step 3 is a further advanced stage of Step 2 and is intended to convey "Kisoku" from the upper half of the body to the leg (KI-1) of the lower half of the body. Emphasis in this Step 3 is put on a much thinner and longer respiration. At inspiration, the lower teeth ridge is touched by the tongue with the mouth slightly open and "Ki" is made to pass through the abdomen with the abdomen expanded accordingly. Then, "Ki" is made to reach CV-1, wherefrom it is led to both legs along the outside of the thigh and finally to KI-1. When inhaling, the abdominal region is gradually compressed. "Ki" is raised from KI-1 with the upper teeth touched by the tongue and is gathered at CV-1 by raising it again along the inside of both legs. Then, it is made to raise through the anus and up to the GV-20 through the coccygeal vertebra, the backbone and the cervical nape. Further, "Ki" is divided into two at the front side of both ears and follows down along both cheeks to the tip of the tongue so as to contact "Kisoku" at respiration.

As a stance for exercising Step 3, a "Form of Three Circles" or a "Form of Three Matches" in the erect position is recommended. When exhaling, relax yourself and lower the body in line with the progress of "Ki." The stance in this exercise is linked to the pose of a big bird with its lower body pulled back which

Fig. 51

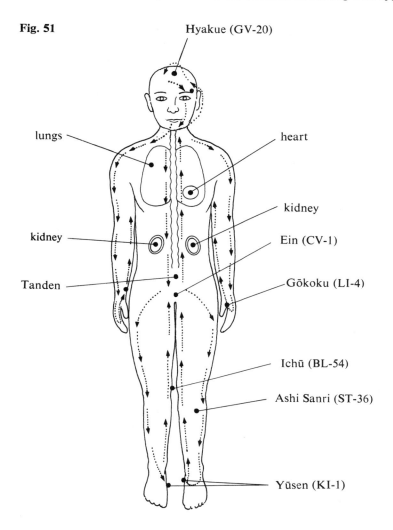

Hyakue (GV-20)

lungs

heart

kidney

kidney

Ein (CV-1)

Tanden

Gōkoku (LI-4)

Ichū (BL-54)

Ashi Sanri (ST-36)

Yūsen (KI-1)

is about to fly.

When inhaling, take up a stance in such a way that the toes grip the ground similarly to a large tree taking root firmly in the ground.

The most appropriate time for exercising Step 3 is when the sun begins to rise in the east. First, face the sun and close both eyes to harmonize the breathing with the light of the sun. Concentrate the whole mind on obtaining a state of mind in which "the sun," "human being" and "Ki" form a trinity. Step 3 is the most important of all Steps from 1 through 6. For adjustment of "Kisoku" in the exercise of Step 3, therefore, especially severe conditions are called for; for example, a soundless, uniform and continued breathing are imposed.

Inspiration and expiration must be a thin breath barely felt, which is called "Shinsoku." A respiration involving sound is called "Fusoku," a soundless but not so thin respiration, "Kisoku" and stagnated respiration, "Zesoku." Unlike "shinsoku" required in Step 3, these breathing methods cannot be said to be desirable breathing methods for exercises.

The reason why the breathing method in this Step 3 is more important than other methods is that it has a favorable effect not only on the cure of diseases and maintenance of health, but also on the nervous systems. In particular, it is important in that it eliminates a congestion of the central nerve and the brain and strengthens each organ of the human body. This breathing method promotes a reflex action of the nerve center as well as the spinal cord and stimulates peripheral nerves of the entire body to remedy the causes of diseases in the body.

Therefore, by exercising Step 3 for about six months, it is possible to lower high blood pressure and cure chronic diseases such as nervous prostration, insomnia, heart disease, arteriosclerosis and menstrual irregularity.

Step 4 (Back to the pattern of natural breathing)

This type of breathing, as in the case of normal respiration, belongs to the same pattern as that shown in Step 1, while it differs from those shown in Steps 2 and 3. There is, however, little difference between Steps 1 and 4. The breathing described in Step 4 emphasizes extension to both extremes of tension and relaxation. This pattern of respiration is called the "natural abdominal breathing." In this pattern of breathing, the abdominal region is contracted while exhaling, and expanded while inhaling.

While undergoing Step 4 breathing exercise, it is appropriate to stand in a posture called "Form of Three Circles" or "Form of Three Matches." Similar movements as those for Steps 2 and 3 are used. The "Unki (breathing works)," however, must be carried out in accordance with the nature of the patient's health.

This normal abdominal respiration exercise follows two consecutive reversal abdominal respiration exercises (Steps 2 and 3). This is because patients suffering from conditions such as hypertension suffer strains in their respiration process after undergoing Steps 1 and 2 exercises. It is necessary to condition back to normal abdominal respiration through ten minutes of the Step 4 exercise in order to relay the respiratory system.

This form of respiration helps activate the lower abdominal muscles and accelerate vertical movements of the diaphragm. As a result, it strengthens the abdominal muscle for respiratory purposes and controls and adjusts abnormalities in the functions of digestive organs such as stomach, liver, intestines and pancreas. It is therefore helpful for those recuperating from chronic diseases such as gastric ptosis, peptic ulcer and duodenal ulcer. Furthermore, this type of breathing exercise is beneficial in the treatment of serious diseases such as phthisis, bronchial asthma, and heart failure. This is because it helps overcome difficulties caused by dyspnea which in turn results from ailment of lungs and bronchial tubes.

It has been proven that this pattern of respiration is successful in the treatment of those recuperating from diseases in the digestive organs, such as enteritis, enteroparesis, liver trouble, gallstones, renal calculosis and menstrual irregularities. This is because functions of the various digestive organs are activated due to the exaggerated vertical motion of the diaphragm and abdominal muscles. This patttern of breathing exercise also helps control the performance of various digestive organs and secretion of digestive juice and enzymes. It is also capable of having considerable effects in the cure of chronic diseases in the respiratory organs.

Step 5 (Involves a breathing exercise to maintain health and immunity to various illnesses)

This method is designed to reinforce the effects of Steps 1 and 2 breathing exercises. It is thus necessary for the patients to have learned the breathing exercises described in Steps 1 to 4 completely before going into this Step 5. The four preceding breathing exercises help the patients to recover from various illnesses. The Step 5 exercise is said to reinforce the recovery.

The Step 5 exercise is to be carried out in the same way as in Step 2. The only point that differs from it is that the mouth and nasal cavity should be narrowed and the vocal fold stiffened. Efforts should be made to take small, light breaths smoothly and consecutively. They are to be taken in a similar pattern as that of "Shinsoku." The abdominal respiration must be exaggerated to the extreme. The exaggeration results in accelerated expanding and contracting movements for the abdomen.

The main purpose of this exercise is to further strengthen the functions and nerves of the body from what one has already been in training for several months through the vigorous exercises of Steps 2, 3 and 4. The Step 5 exercise is designed to have considerable effects in upkeeping prolonged and healthy lives.

The postures taken in performing this exercise are the "Form of Three Circles," "Form of Three Matches" and "Form of Holding a Tiger Down." One should sit squarely, or quietly, or must lie down on the back or on the side to carry out this step. The exercise is to be conducted continuously for three months before proceeding to the next step, the concluding Step 6.

Step 6 (Thoracic respiration no longer used, and navel used for taking breaths)

This breathing exercise is considered the most important of those innovated in the Orient. It is generally said that it would take at least several years of rigorous training to prepare a patient for this important exercise.

The main purpose of the Step 6 exercise is the maintenance of health and age. This breathing method is characterized by the formal breathing pattern called the "Shinsoku." Taking the "Shinsoku" instills the root and extends the span of human life. The "Shinsoku" breathing starts with the controlling of the breath. The heart must be calmed and the mouth shut. When undergoing the exercise in the morning, it is necessary to stand. In the evening, one must be seated. This would bring about the best results.

The exercise should be performed according to the urethra method described Step 3. First, posture oneself in the right style and calm the heart and the body. It is therefore necessary to regulate both the mind and the breathing so that the movement and inactivity can be harmonized. Counting while breathing will help tranquilize the heart over a certain period.

Next, one must move on to "Zuisoku" and start taking in normal breaths as one does unconsciously. In doing this, each breath becomes thinner and longer. By and by, it becomes relaxed and natural. Outwardly, the respiration would seem

Fig. 52

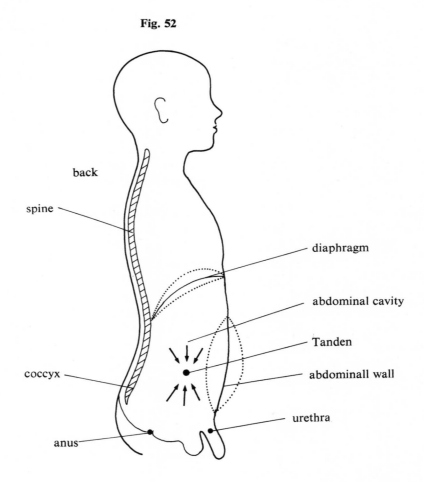

It is absolutely necessary to harmonize the mind and the body: first concentrate on your lower abdominal region in the Tanden. Then exhale with the tongue automatically touching the lower gum while the abdominal section of the body is expanded. When inhaling, the tongue must touch the upper gum and the abdominal section must be contracted.

to have stopped completely. This state is called the "Musoku (state of breathless-ness)." While in this state, the mind must be concentrated on "Naikan" (inner reflection) while the "Sokusō" (aspects of the breath taken) should attain the eight standards of "Yū" (calm), "Kan" (easing), "Sai" (thinness), "Kin" (uni-formity), "Sei" (inactivity), "Nan" (softness), "Shin" (depth), and "Chō" (length).

In shifting from the state of "Zuisoku" (natural breathing) to that of "Musoku" (breathlessness), apparent changes will take place in the states of the mind and the body. In experiencing these changes, the "Ki" which has been controlling the movements of various parts of the body consciously, will start to control them unconsciously.

For those entering this state of unconscious stability, spontaneous vibrations are felt in the mind and the body while exhaling. Also, a heated sensation will be felt in the center of the lower abdomen as it moves to the soft spot near the anus and finally to the sole of the foot. The heat will then start to circulate through all parts of the body. This situation establishes an inner communication throughout the entire body. The body thus feels instilled by energy in such a way that the body seems to expand endlessly from one's room to the entire city, and then into infinite corners of space.

Those who successfully experience this state would appear to be sitting, or standing as the case might be, in a state of complete calmness and unconscious-ness. Internally, however, their internal world would be undergoing drastic changes. The secret principle of the state of "Shinsoku," therefore, is that upon mastering the true breath, one can attain the delicate mental situation leading to the religious awakening called "Satori" in Buddhism. This spiritual awakening is based on the idea that all things existing in this world should be as they are under the holy teaching of Buddha. No thing existing in this world should deny its own vitality. Therefore, the state of "Musoku" is said to lead one's mind to attain the highest perception of "Nehan" (Buddhahood, or supreme enlighten-ment) in Buddhist philosophy.

As mentioned before, the "correct" method of respiration innovated in the practice of Oriental medicine is divided into two parts. The first comprises the breathing patterns described in Steps 1 to 4, and the second those described in Steps 5 and 6. Those in the first group are beneficial in the process of recuperation from illnesses as well as for the maintenance of the health. The purpose for those in the second group transcends mere recuperation and extends into the prolong-ment of life. The latter group is thus said to be characterized by philosophical meditation which is believed to be the best way to extend life span.

Needless to say, people have to make utmost efforts in order to achieve ultimate long life. However, reminder must be made to those suffering from present illness to exert their entire efforts to master the basic breathing exercises (Steps 1 to 4) so that they are able to recover fully back to health.

In other words, Steps 5 and 6 are designed to impart the end purposes of human life, namely the prolongation of life. This then means that all must concentrate their efforts in achieving this ultimate aim to live better and to live longer.

4. *Reinforcing What Has Been Achieved by the Breathing Exercises*

Auxiliary Breathing Exercises

The respiration exercises are aimed at activating the functions of internal organs within the body. In order to maintain the balance of the body both internally and externally, it is necessary to carry out certain physical exercises. These exercises are for relaxation by extending and contracting the muscles repeatedly.

This physical training is called "Auxiliary Breathing Exercises." In fact, it is vital that it be incorporated into a total program along with the breathing exercises. Introduced here will be ten auxiliary exercises to be performed in parallel with the breathing exercises. It is recommended that those performed in order to improve the particular function of a particular organ be carried out independently from those with other purposes. It is also advised that a couple of these auxiliary exercises, rather than all of the ten, be performed at once. That a patient carries out intensively a couple of them which seem to interest him is suggested.

The main goal of these auxiliary exercises is to upgrade the results of the breathing exercises. They are to be performed immediately before or immediately after undergoing the breathing exercises. These exercises are very beneficial in strengthening the functions of muscles, bones, joints and various organs of the body.

Tapping the abdomen (effective to relax muscles and relieve fatigue)

This training is designed to relax muscles and relieve fatigue. It is therefore advisable to perform this exercise immediately after the breathing exercises. In this exercise, the stomach is massaged with the palm of the hand. This is to ease the tense muscles and improve the circulation of the blood within the body. The massaging aids those suffering constipation while it controls the functions of the intestines.

Methods: First, stand with both feet shoulder width apart. There is no need to intentionally keep the backbone erect. Put one palm on your belly, with the thumb placed on the navel. The other palm should be placed on the indented part of the back. Move both palms vertically and simultaneously upon the abdomen and the back (Fig. 53). Repeat thirty times. Change the hands and massage

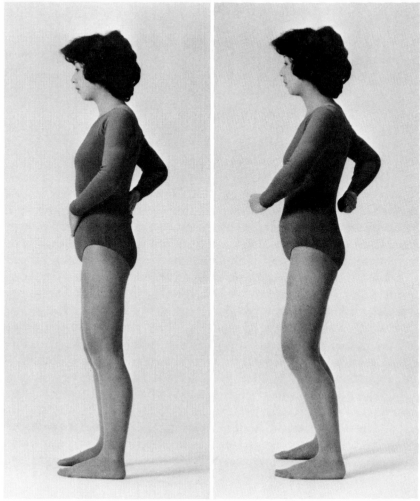

Fig. 53   Fig. 54

in the same manner. Repeat thirty times again. Next, move both palms horizontally and massage thoroughly all around the body at the heigh of the belly in vertical motion. In doing this, one palm must be placed on the front while the other palm is on the back, and massage the front and back simultaneously. Repeat thirty times. Next, with both hands making fists, tap the belly and the back simultaneously, and then move to both sides alternately tapping in the same manner. It is suggested that the knees be bent lightly and shaked with each tap in order to keep a rhythm. This should be repeated more than hundred times (Fig. 54). Change hands again and repeat.

Finally, return to massaging the belly and the back and then both sides in exactly the same way as before.

Yajirobei **exercise**

This exercise is designed to be very effective in the recovery of those suffering from hypertension and heart diseases. This is because it is believed to lower the blood pressure and stabilize the function of the heart.

Methods: First stand with both feet apart a little more than shoulder width, or about 50 centimeters. Both arms are held out horizontally with the palms turned up (Fig. 55). While exhaling from the nose, lean the upper part of the body slowly to the left (Fig. 56). In doing so, the face faces the front and both arms must be held out. When the entire breath is exhaled, the upper body is fixed at this pose. Holding the breath, count from one to three. Then inhale slowly from nose and lift the upper body up vertically. The body is thus returned to the original upright posture. It is necessary, in this exercise, to coordinate the movements of the body and respiration. Next, repeat the same movement but toward the right. Both movements to the right and to the left should be repeated at least thirty times.

Fig. 55 **Fig. 56**

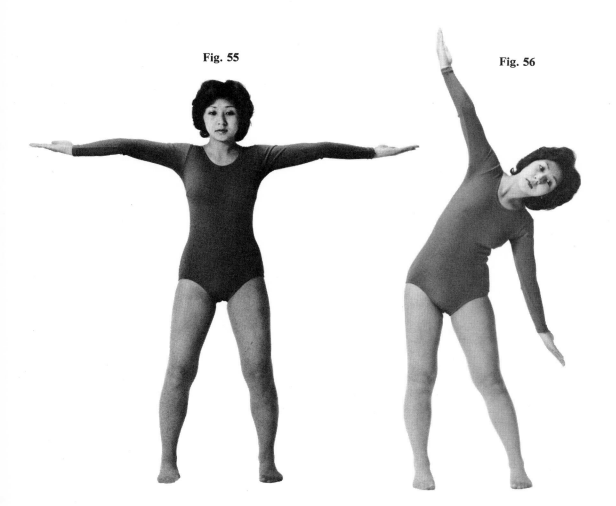

Exercise for twisting the body using waist and feet (to promote activities of stomach and intestines)

This exercise is designed to soften the joints of the body and strengthen all the muscles of the hands, legs and waist. It is also believed to strengthen the digestive organs, especially the stomach and intestines. It is by no means unusual to let wind and belch while undergoing this exercise. This proves that the practice has activated the functions of the stomach and intestines because gases contained therein are freed.

It should be noted, however, that this exercise is not recommended for those suffering from hypertension and heart diseases, because it eventually gives rise to hard pressure against the lower abdomen and often incurs valsalva breath holding. Therefore, it is recommended that those suffering from heart disease and hypertension should take other types of exercise in order to improve their health. Only after recognizing a sufficient improvement in physical condition, should this type of exercise be undertaken.

Fig. 57

Fig. 58

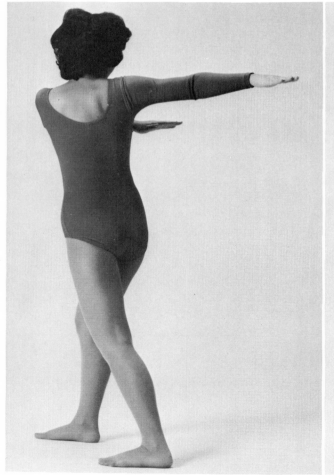
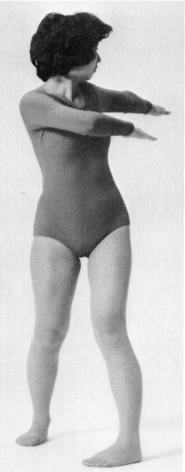

Methods: Open feet wide, separated by about 80–90 centimeters, then squat down in order to assume the posture of riding horseback. In this posture, twist the body alternately to right and left with a spring of the waist and feet and arms held straight out parallel to the ground and following the motion of the body (Figs. 57 and 58). The body weight must be rested alternately on the right and left foot. As an example, if the weight is rested on the left foot, then the body is twisted to the left with both arms following to leftward. The movement of the arms describes the arc of a half circle with the shoulders in the center when the body is turned to the side. Bear in mind that the upper arms do not rise above the level of the shoulder when the arms are swung. This effectively means that when the body is twisted to the left, the left arm has to be held below the level of the left shoulder. The face has to be turned to the left and right alternately in company with the movement of the upper body and arms, and the eyes should follow the movement of the fingers when they move in the line of arc.

The heel of the foot must be slightly raised, not bearing the weight of the body. It is important to maintain a good breathing rhythm while the body is being twisted.

Exercise for shaking the body

This exercise is designed to strengthen the waist and hips, and is believed to assist in recovery from nervous prostration and other types of nervous break-downs. It is recommended, therefore, that those suffering from arthritis, hernia of the intervertebral disc and other diseases related to the joints of the waist should undergo this exercise.

This type of physical exercise is also effective in lowering high blood pressure, normalizing heart activity and activating the functions of the central nervous system.

Methods: The arms are hung away from the sides of the body and relaxed for a while. At first, twist the upper body to the left as much as possible while ex-haling through the nose (Fig. 59). In company with this movement, the whole of the upper body including face, arms, and waist, is to be correspondingly twisted to the left. At this point, remember to keep the palm of the forward hand around the lower abdomen. The heels of both feet have to be placed firmly on the floor, and must not be raised. After exhaling, it is important that having twisted the upper body backward as much as possible you should be able to see the back of the heels. After exhaling through the nose, quietly breathe in, again through nose, while swinging the upper body back to the previous position.

It is very important in this exercise to remember to have the movement of the upper body in phase with your breathing cycle, so that when inspiration is com-pleted, the movement of the upper body is halted with full-face turned to the front.

Next, turn the upper body to the right and swing both arms in the same direc-

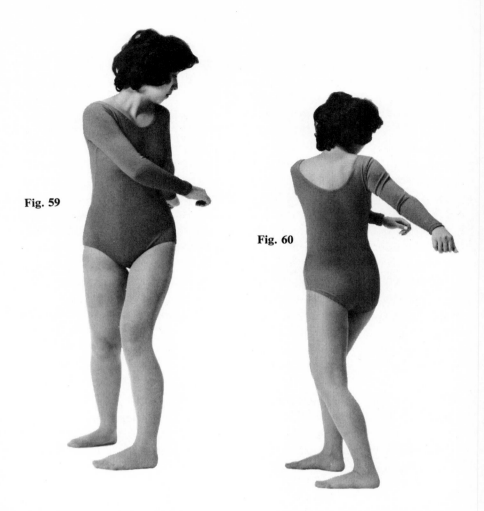

Fig. 59

Fig. 60

tion while slowly exhaling through the nose (Fig. 60). Having twisted the body to the right beyond the point where both heels can be seen, the body's movement must be temporarily stopped and followed by the halting of expiration. Now, swing the body back to the previous position while quietly inhaling through the nose.

Carry out this exercise twisting the body from left to right alternately, remembering that the movement of the upper body must keep in phase with the cycle of breathing. This type of physical exercise is very effective for curing various diseases such as arthritis, hernia of the intervertebral disc, and other ailments associated with the joints. The reason for this is because this exercise is believed to have a beneficial effect on the deep-lying areas of the human body.

Rowing boat exercise

This type of physical exercise is effective for strengthening all the muscles and bones of the body. The movement of the body is very similar to the movements involved while rowing a boat. All the upper and lower parts of the body are used for rowing and should be moved with good timing to ensure the steady movement of the boat. As the rowing exercise is effectively hard training equivalent to that experienced when rowing a boat, it is not recommended for those suffering from hypertension; people with heart diseases are strictly prohibited from taking this exercise.

On the other hand, the effectiveness of this exercise is so great that it will strengthen the functions of those muscles and bones related to the waist and other major parts of the body. All pain felt in joints throughout the body is eliminated while undergoing this exercise. Therefore, it is believed that this exercise is a "youth pill" for rejuvenating people inasmuch as various body cells are stimulated.

Methods: Step forward with the right foot about 70 centimeters. Then, bend the right leg to form a right angle between the lower leg and thigh keeping the kneecap vertically in line with the big toe. The left leg is stretched straight backward and the hips swung toward the right leg. The arms are stretched forward at the level of the shoulders and both hands clenched to make fists (Fig. 61). Start to exhale through the nose while bending the upper body toward the right

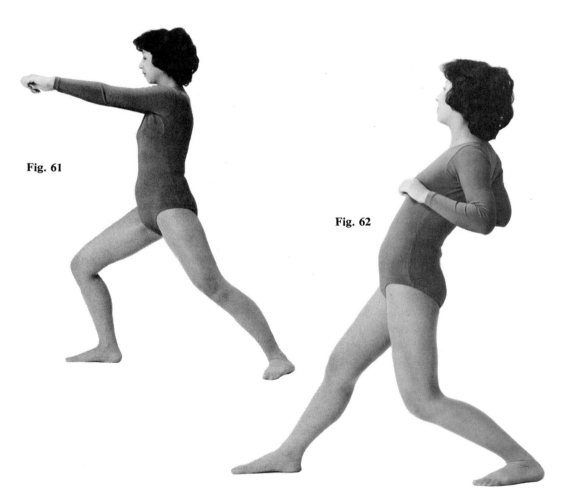

Fig. 61

Fig. 62

leg. Simultaneously stretch both arms forward as with a forward oar stroke. Then, pull back the upper body while quietly inhaling through the nose. Simultaneously, bend both arms, pull them back to the chest, and also bend the upper body backward (Fig. 62).

Remember to keep the movements of the upper body in phase with the breathing cycle, pulling the arms back to the chest before inspiration is completed.

When one round of motion is completed, the right leg which was placed forward is straight and the left leg bent. After repeating the rowing motion nine times together with correct breathing, reverse the leg positions and put the left foot forward, the right foot to the rear. Continue another round of the exercise a further nine times. Carry out thirty full sets of the exercise, each including nine rounds of rowing motion alternately on the right and left legs.

Exercise for carrying a ball

This exercise is believed to be effective for curing lame hips. It is recommended

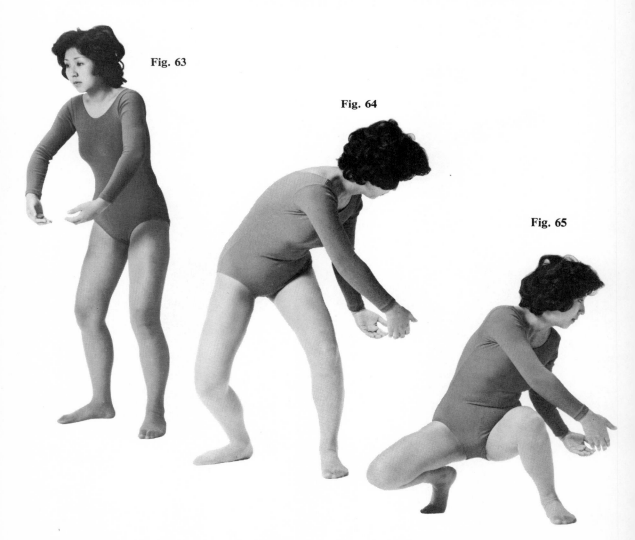

Fig. 63

Fig. 64

Fig. 65

that people who should carry out this type of exercise are those suffering from lumbago and headache resulting from severe lumbago. It is also effective for curing a bend of the waist.

Methods: Keep both legs widely separated with a span of more than 100 centimeters, clench the fists and stretch both arms naturally downward keeping a distance between arms and abdomen of about 60 centimeters (Fig. 63). This posture resembles that of a person carrying a basketball in front of the abdomen. Then, still carrying the imaginary ball, twist the upper body leftward while gradually lowering the left hip (Fig. 64). At that time, exhale through the nose while twisting the upper body. When the body is twisted at right angles to the line linking the feet, a crouching posture is assumed upon completion of expiration (Fig. 65). Remember that the movements of the body must coincide with the various phases of the breathing cycle. When maintaining the posture of squatting on the heels, the upper body should be kept straight, with the spinal column in a straight line. Do not move the upper body from side to side.

After completing expiration, inhale through the nose while turning the body to face forward, and slowly stand up (Figs. 66 and 67). After standing up straight facing forward, inspiration is completed. Remember that inspiration must coincide with the movements of the body. The arms must be swung in the same direction as the body when twisting sideways.

Now, turn the upper body toward the right while slowly crouching down on the heels. Simultaneously, exhale slowly through the nose. When sitting on the heels, expiration is completed. Then, start to slowly inhale through the nose while turning the body to face forward, and raise the body vertically.

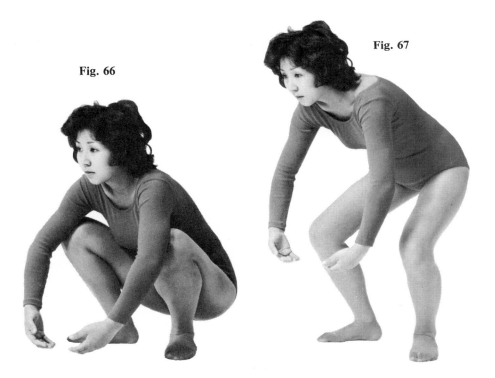

Fig. 66

Fig. 67

Carry out at least nine rounds of the exercise during one session, with each round consisting of twisting the upper body to left and right alternately. It is recommended to carry a basketball while exercising.

If this exercise is carried out as frequently as possible, it is expected that its effectiveness will soon be felt in curing such diseases as lame hip, lumbago, and headache caused by sharp lumbago pains.

Exercise for pulling legs up out of marsh

This exercise is very useful for curing joint pains, arthritis and for recovery from pulmonary tuberculosis and asthma. Additionally, the exercise is very effective for envigorating those people suffering from various intractable diseases.

The type of physical training involved is also believed to be very effective in stimulating the functions of the central nervous system, regulating the respiratory cycle, and alleviating those diseases related to circulatory organs, such as hypertension and heart disease.

Methods: A considerable amount of room is required because exercisers have to move from one point to another during training. First, step forward with the right foot and then draw the left foot backward. Maintain a distance between the feet of about 70 centimeters and an angle of 75 degrees between the legs. Now assume a posture in which the right leg is bent slightly at the knee, the left leg being stretched out behind in a straight line. Clench both hands to make fists and hold them up above the head in front of the forehead (Fig. 68).

In this position, imagine that the fists are being used to support from below a ladder which is standing against a wall. Next, draw the left foot slowly back to the heel of the right foot, while inhaling quietly through the nose (Fig. 69). The rear foot is not raised from the floor when being drawn forward. However act as though you are straining to raise the foot. And try to keep the left leg stretched in a straight line while moving. The other leg set forward must be kept firm as it works as the axis. The whole weight rests on the right foot while moving the other foot. In this motion, the left foot is moved in a way resembling pulling free from imaginary marsh, and is brought to the side of the other foot. When both feet are level, inspiration is completed. Then, start to exhale through the nose while slowly moving the left leg forward. Do not lift the sole of the foot from the surface of the floor.

Next, draw the right foot forward to a position level with the left foot which was previously placed forward. While moving the leg left to the rear, do not bend it at the knee. Then, remember to keep the movement of the foot in phase with inspiration. The breathing cycle comes to an end when the foot movement is completed.

In other words, hold up both hands in a way resembling supporting a ladder from below, then shuffle forward across the floor. This type of movement with the feet sliding over the floor surface is often used in Judo.

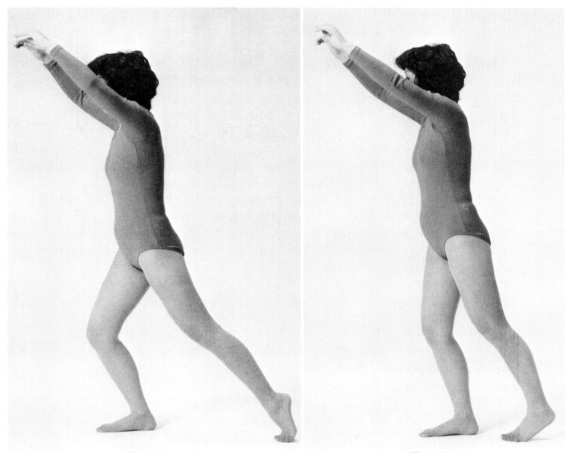

Fig. 68   Fig. 69

The key point of this exercise is to inhale through the nose, instead of exhaling, at the beginning of physical training. Other types of exercise start with expiration instead of inspiration.

Exercise in *Sumo* crouching posture

This exercise is very useful for recovering expended energy and is believed to have a beneficial effect in strengthening the muscles of arms and legs and the joints of all parts of the body, especially both sides of the waist. It is helpful for replenishing spent Tanden and strengthening the movements of hands and legs. In Oriental medicine, Tanden, the center of the abdominal region, is believed to be a key spot where the energy of mental and physical activity is concentrated. For this reason it is said that any physical training which is able to stimulate this part of the body may help extend the life span. In this regard this exercise is said to be greatly beneficial in recuperating from various diseases.

It should be remembered that those people suffering from heart disease, asthma or hypertension are strictly forbidden to take this exercise.

Methods: Assume a standing posture with both feet level and opened slightly wider than shoulder width (Fig. 70). The distance between the feet should be about 50 centimeters. Both arms are raised forward at shoulder level and curved inward to make a big circle similar to the posture shown in "Forms of the Three Circles." Clench the fists. Then, exhale from the nose slowly and crouch down on the heels while keeping the posture of the upper body unchanged. While squatting down on the hams, the hips are dropped between the heels of both feet. In this case do not allow the upper body to fall forward or lean forward. Both heels should be kept firmly on the floor throughout this exercise. Having exhaled through the nose, crouch down low to the floor and touch the floor with both fists (Fig. 71). Then, inhale from the nose slowly, raise the fists from the floor and stand up vertically. Both arms are simultaneously gradually lifted from the lower part of the abdominal region to shoulder height. Having completed inspiration, return to the former posture of standing straight, with the arms held at shoulder heigh. Then, beginning to slowly exhale, start to crouch down on the heels.

Repeat this round of physical exercise which is similar to the preparatory windup for *sumo* wrestlers', five times for calisthenics training. Then, having exhaled through the nose, stretch the arms forward and raise the upper body while keeping the form of squatting down on the hams, slowly inhale through the nose. After completing inspiration, pull back the arms to the body bending at elbow, then open the forearms and hands outward as wide as possible. Having opened out the forearms and hands, bring them together in front of the chest and clap both hands (Fig. 72), while vigorously exhaling through the nose. After clapping the hands, quickly inhale through the nose while opening out the forearms and hands in a quick motion. Having completed inspiration, exhale through the nose while bringing the hands together in front of the chest, and clap hands in a single breath. Concentrate all strength from all parts of the body into the abdominal region while clapping the hands. Repeat this round of exercise five times continuously. Then inhale while stretching the arms forward. After completing inspiration exhale through the nose, putting the arms behind your back and vigorously clap hands in the rear, slightly raising the body on the heels while keeping the backbone straight. Now, open out the arms while inhaling through the nose. On completion of inspiration, clap hands behind your back while exhaling rapidly through the nose.

Repeat this exercise five times. With the completion of five rounds of each exercise, full sets of this exercise are completed. It is recommended that people of delicate build carry out the exercise with the help of a support such as a desk, table, etc. For instance, while carrying out the exercise for squatting down on the heels and standing up vertically, place the hands on a desk or dining table in order to keep the body upright. This practice is said to reduce the effectiveness to the exercises, but is nevertheless still recommendable to accustom those of delicate build to this exercise. Remember not to put strength into the arms while

Fig. 70   Fig. 71

Fig. 72

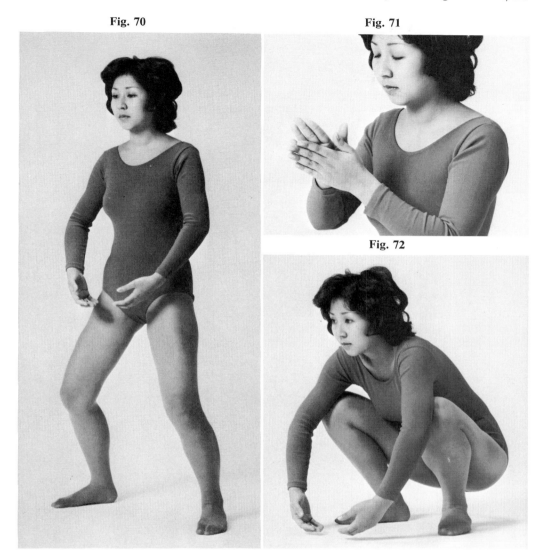

they are being used to balance the upper body during the exercise.

Physical exercise with bar

This exercise is said to be very beneficial for eliminating fatigue, making the muscles more supple and for accelerating the rate of blood flow throughout the body. It is also believed to have some effect in calming the functions of the brain after being in a high state of activity, and in envigorating the working of the entire body.

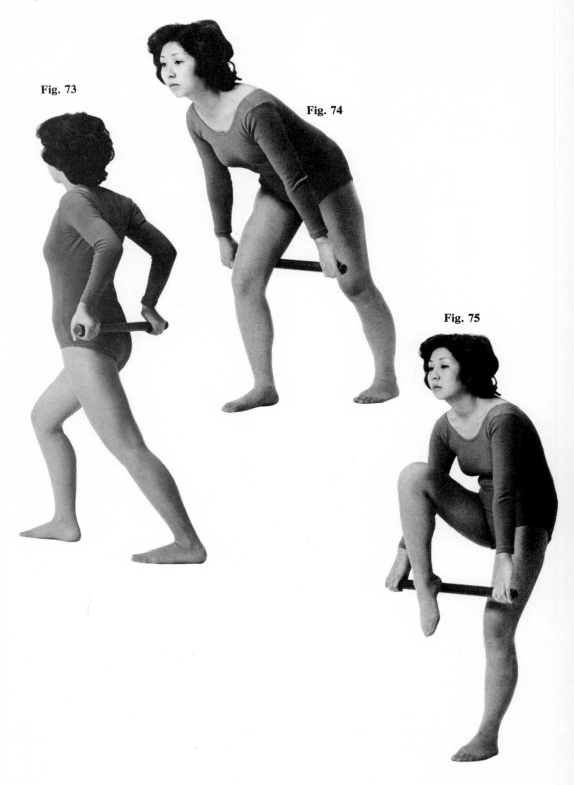

Fig. 73

Fig. 74

Fig. 75

Methods: Obtain a bar with a length of some 50 centimeters—any bar like a golf club shaft or the plastic tubing accompanying a vacuum cleaner can be used for this exercise.

Grip the bar lightly with both hands, and stand in the "Form of Three Circles." Hold the bar in front of the upper body, and gradually lift it up above the head while slowly inhaling through the nose. After taking air into the lungs through the nose, lift the bar over the head to the rear, and "scrub" the back, waist, buttocks and back of the legs with the bar (Fig. 73). While exhaling through the nose, pass the bar to the front by stepping over it (Figs. 74 and 75). After doing so, hold the breath for a while and return to the initial posture. Repeat this round of the exercise seven times. Then, while inhaling through the nose, lower the bar and pass it to the rear by stepping over it. While slowly exhaling through the nose, rub the back of the legs, buttocks, hips, and back with the bar, moving from bottom to top.

Remember that the movements of the bar should coincide with the phases of the respiratory cycle; for instance, complete expiration when the bar reaches the top of the head after finishing the scrubbing procedure. While holding the breath, slowly bring the bar back to the front of the body to the initial position.

Repeat this round of exercise seven times continuously. It is also recommended to carry out this exercise constantly in combination with the other type of exercise utilizing the bar; for instance, massage the whole of the body with the bar swinging around, scrubbing and kneading the body.

Rhythmical exercise

This exercise is believed to have a definite effect in banishing fatigue, relieving tension built up in the body and in easing the movements of muscles and bones. An overactive brain center is rapidly calmed on proper performance of the exercise. Therefore, it is believed that this exercise is very useful for winding down the mind and body after undergoing hard physical and/or mental activity such as book reading, sports training, and other types of physical and mental work.

Methods: Stand with the feet level and at shoulder width apart. Then, raise the heel of the right foot, placing the big toe of the right foot and the heel of the left foot firmly on the floor. Then, raise the right hand above the head, and thrust it firmly upward with the index finger stretched out and the other four fingers bent naturally (Fig. 76). Rest the whole of the body weight on the left foot and rhythmically move the body up and down using the right foot as a spring. The more the body is moved in this exercise, the greater the benefit derived. Therefore, remember to move the upper body rhythmically to musical accompaniment where possible. The body must be moved forward, backward, and to the left and right in company with the music.

Having bounced about 40–50 times, change feet and hands. This time, the weight of the body is rested on the right foot, while the heel of the left foot is

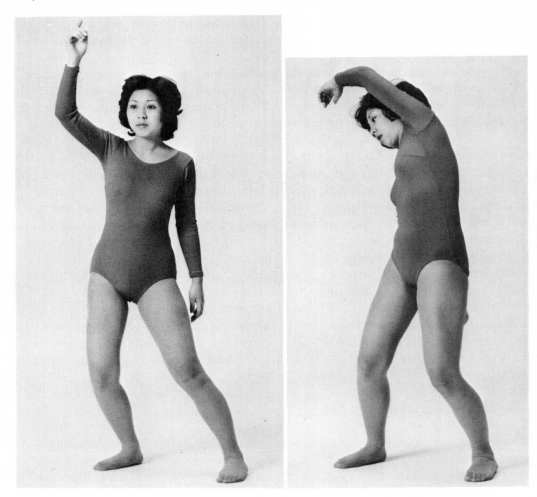

Fig. 76   **Fig. 77**

raised to jerk the body backward and forward as well as to left and right. The left hand is raised above the head to lead the rhythmical movement of the body. Repeat more than 40–50 times in one set of exercise. Then, holding both hands upward simultaneously continue to complete a set of exercise. After doing so, bring the arms to the side of the body, relax, and shake the upper body with the hands moving loosely (Fig. 77).

These patterns of exercises discussed above are all auxiliary body exercises designed to promote further the effectiveness of breathing exercises. Such auxiliary exercises are introduced in this chapter to enable you to select two of your own choice, bearing in mind their individual merits. Therefore, it is not necessary to master the secrets of all these auxiliary exercises. It is better to pick only those which are most comfortable and beneficial to you, after thoroughly trying out all the exercises. You should also make your selection with due regard to your physical condition and any disease from which you might be suffering.

Among the ten patterns of exercises introduced in this chapter it is firmly advised that four major exercises should be carried out without fail each time after carrying out the breathing exercises, because such auxiliary exercises are designed to ease tension built up from undergoing the breathing exercises and to relieve fatigue.

The four recommended exercises are Tapping the Abdomen, Twisting the Upper Body, Shaking the Upper Body and the Bar Exercise. The remaining six exercises have been proven sufficiently efficacious for improving health even when carried out separately from the breathing exercises.

It is not recommended for the Rhythmical Exercises to be conducted in a dusty or crowded place such as a dance floor or disco. Taking into consideration the beneficial effect on health of these exercises, they should be carried out in quiet and clean surroundings, such as a gymnasium, public hall or park.

Before taking these exercises it is advised to refrain from taking alcoholic beverages or other stimulants in order to maintain good physical condition.

Five Stances Designed to Promote the Effectiveness of Breathing Exercises

The following five stances resemble those common to five different kinds of animals and enable one to enjoy longevity as they are designed to further promote the effectiveness of breathing exercises. They were derived some 2,000 years ago from Oriental medicine for the purpose of helping people realize eternal youth, long life, strong physique and preservation of health. All are designed to assist in recovery from diseases and for encouraging the motions of the limbs, and it is therefore recommendable to practice regularly every day in order to obtain the full benefit of the breathing exercises. Even if you feel languid and fatigued, do not allow yourself to be overcome by feelings of apathy. Stir your mind to tide over laziness by purposefully carrying out these exercises until you start to perspire. After breaking into a sweat, you should feel refreshed both in mind and body.

Tiger stance

Place your hands and feet flat on the floor and get down on all fours with the back arched and buttocks pointing upward. Then, jump forward and backward (Fig. 78). Do this fourteen times at first (seven forward jumps and seven backward jumps). Then, place your legs to the rear to assume the posture of push-ups (Fig. 79). Gradually lower your abdomen to the floor and thrust out your chest, throwing the head backward (Fig. 80) and looking vertically upward; then return to the initial posture. Do this exercise fourteen times at first.

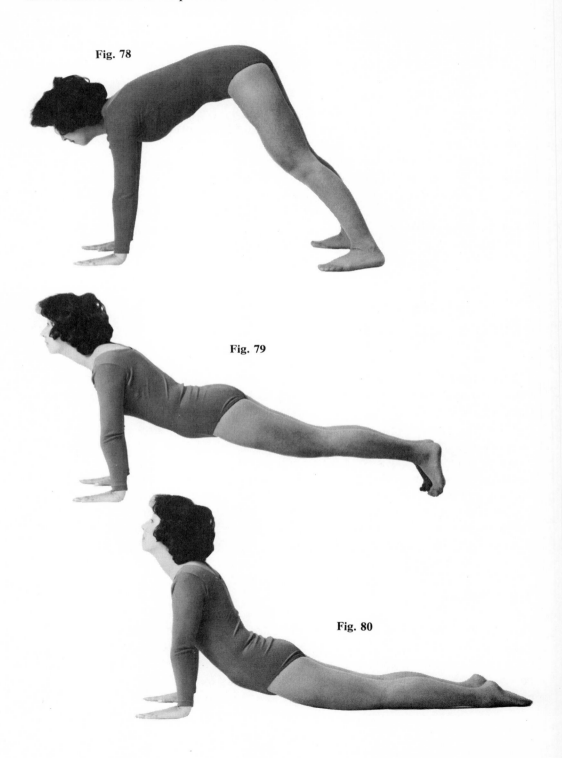

Fig. 78

Fig. 79

Fig. 80

Deer stance

Place your hands and feet flat on the floor and throw back your head. Then, turn your head to the left three times and to the right three times alternately (Fig. 81). Kick back each leg alternately and stretch the leg in a straight line. Carry out this exercise seven times (Fig. 82).

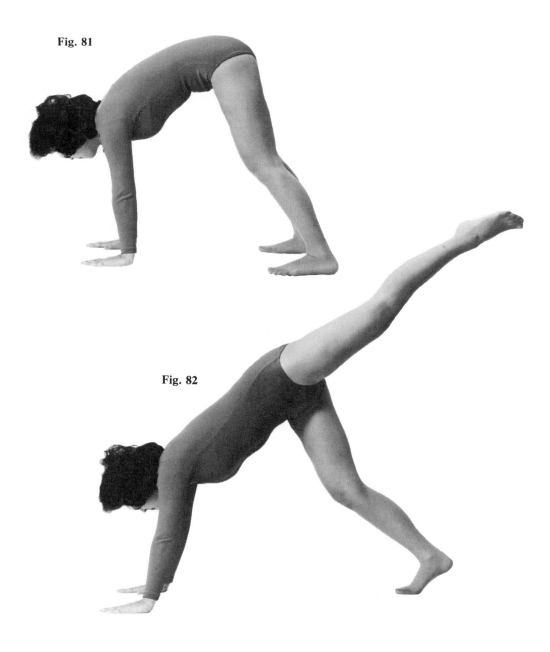

Fig. 81

Fig. 82

Bear stance

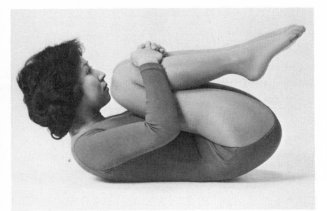

Lie down on your back on the floor and tightly clasp the knees to your chest, holding them with both arms and with the head held up (Fig. 83). Then, roll to the left seven times, followed by rolling to the right seven times (Fig. 84). Kneel down and place your forehead against the floor, stretching your arms over the head.

Fig. 83

Fig. 84

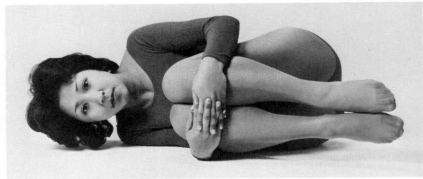

Monkey stance

Carry out chin-ups using an iron bar or tree branch seventeen times (Fig. 85). Then, hang from the bar or branch with both knees hooked over it. Swing your body seven times while hanging, hands gripping the bar and both arms stretched straight (Fig. 86).

Release the hands from the bar and hold the back of the neck with them. Rotate your head seven times while remaining in this position.

Bird stance

Stand on one leg, and bend the waist to lean the upper body forward parallel to the floor. Open both arms wide to 180 degrees and stretch the other leg backward; the rear leg and the arms should be kept at the same level as the upper body and parallel to the floor (Fig. 87). (Assume a posture that a ballerina might assume in "Swan Lake.") Remember to throw your face upward, turn the head to left and right alternately, and move all muscles in the face simultaneously. Then, move the arms further round toward the back without bending the elbows, thus bringing the shoulder blades together (Fig. 88).

Fig. 85

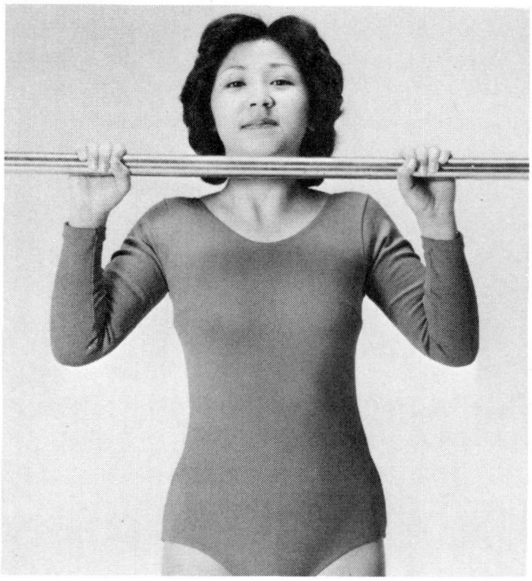

Fig. 86

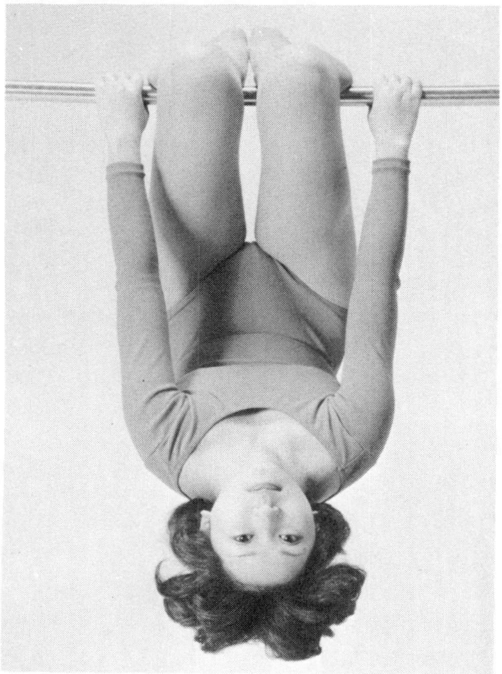

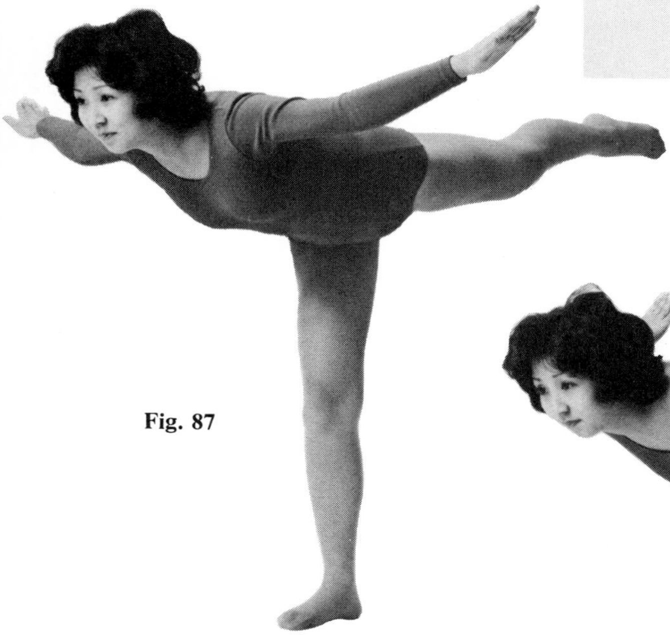

Fig. 87

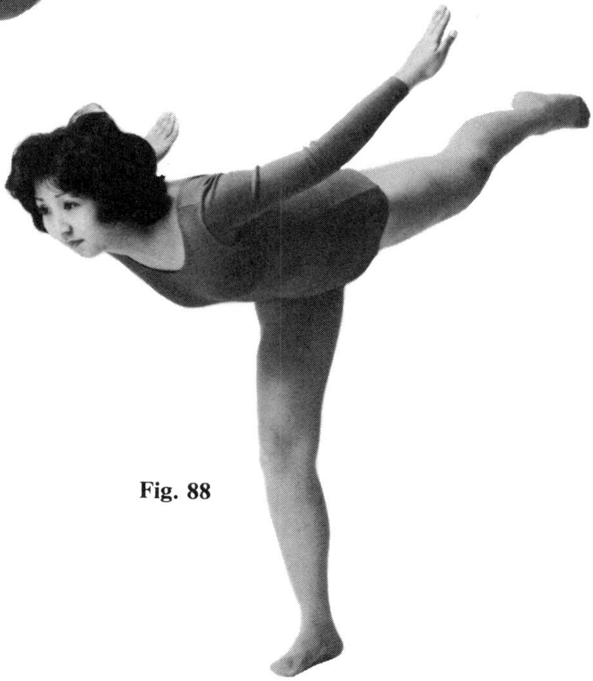

Fig. 88

Fig. 89

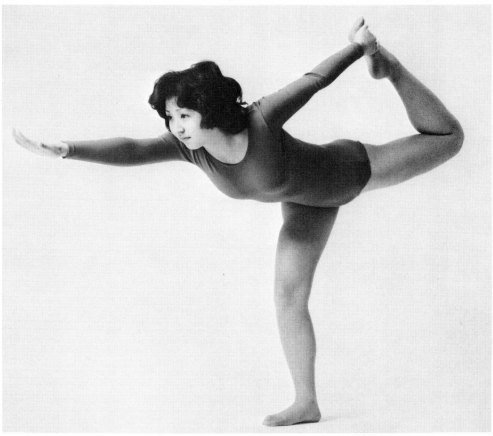

Then, lift up the upper body and thrust forward the leg which had been stretched backward. Lower the hips as much as possible. Holding the forward leg straight, massage it with both hands from thigh to the tip of the toe. After completing this, change leg and repeat the exercise. Repeat this exercise seven times for each leg.

Having done this, returning to the initial position, bend the knee of the leg stretched backward, and grip the instep of the foot with the hand on the same side of the body. Stretch the other hand straight forward parallel to the ground and look down the length of the arm to the tips of the fingers of the hand stretched forward (Fig. 89).

Repeat this exercise for as long as possible. Then, return to the natural posture, and massage the length and breadth of the body with both hands. The above-mentioned stance is the bird stance. These exercises in animal stances must be continued until breaking into a sweat. After starting to perspire, rub your body with hot towels. If you practice regularly over a considerable period of time, you should be able to avoid various kinds of diseases, and regain youthfulness, have a long life and strong physique. Remember to practice slowly and calmly and to control your breathing while undergoing this exercise.

Massage and Shiatsu

Respiration activates the human body through the effect on the internal organs. But martial arts, sports, the auxiliary exercises previously mentioned, and exercises in animal postures exert their effect from the outside. Massage, shiatsu, acupuncture and moxibustion also exert their effect on the body from the exterior, and are designed to assist in recovery from diseases and to recover the strength of the body.

There are certain distinctions which can be made between the group consisting of martial arts, sports and auxiliary exercises and the group comprising massage and moxibustion in their ways of inducing spirit in patients. The former group has a general influence throughout the body, while the latter stimulates a particular part or organ of the body.

Oriental massage consists of six major practical methods as follows:

1. *Keisatsu* method (Light rubbing method)
2. *Jūnetsu* method (Soft kneading method)
3. *Annetsu* method (Squeezing and kneading method)
4. *Appaku* method (Pressure method)
5. *Kōda* method (Tapping method)
6. *Shinsen* method (Vibration method)

The *Keisatsu* method is said to be the most popular massage practice among the Japanese. First, lightly press the palm to the skin and rub up and down and to the left and right while maintaining a constant pressure (Fig. 90). The secret of this light rubbing massage method is to hold the fingers together straight out and to keep the palm and fingers flat.

The *Jūnetsu* method is mainly used for massaging muscles throughout the body. The area to be massaged is firmly held, and the motion of the arm is also employed in effecting the massage (Fig. 91).

Fig. 90   **Fig. 91**

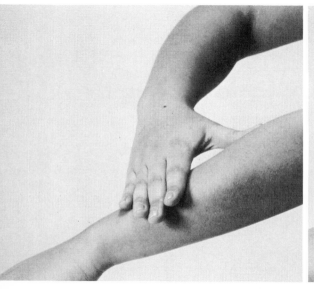
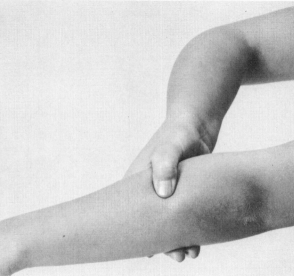

The *Annetsu* method is a massage technique using one or two fingers to massage the joints and bones which should be treated with other connecting parts by pressing the middle finger or the thumb vertically onto the affected area. Gradually increase pressure while describing a circle (Figs. 92 and 93).

The *Appaku* method is a massage technique for applying pressure to the surface of the body with the palm or thumb, or the four fingers together. The palm and fingers are gradually moved from the limb extremities inward (Figs. 94 and 95). The pressure involved is estimated to average about 5–6 kilograms per square centimeter and must be applied to coincide with expiration.

Fig. 92   **Fig. 93**

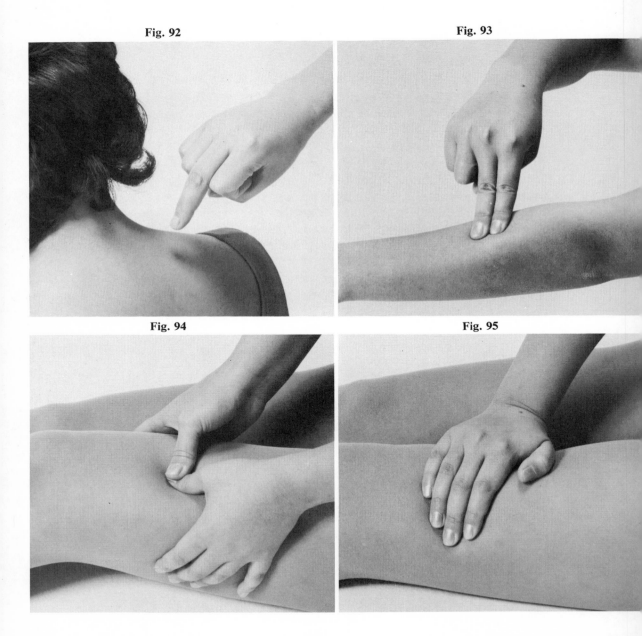

Fig. 94   **Fig. 95**

Fig. 96

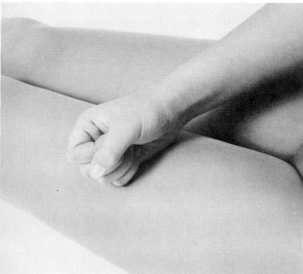

Fig. 97

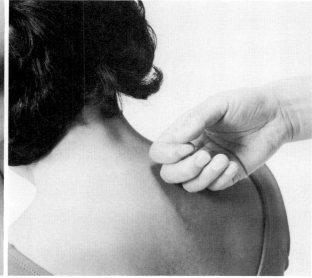

Fig. 98

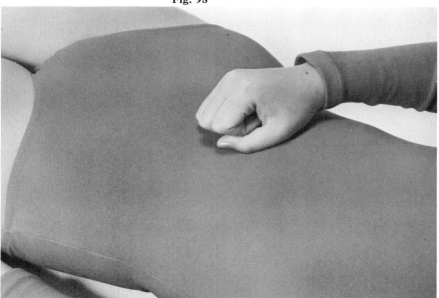

The *Kōda* method is a technique for tapping the affected parts of the body with the little-finger side of the fist (Figs. 96 and 97). Place one of the palms on areas which may be painful due to excess stiffness or areas with activated nervous systems, and rhythmically tap over it with the fist of the other hand.

When dealing with the abdominal region, lightly pat with the inside of the fist (Fig. 98). When tapping a soft part of the body, it may be found better to lightly tap with the side of the hand (Figs. 99 and 100).

The *Shinsen* method is a technique for helping to restore the function of damaged areas of the peripheral nervous system and muscles, the fingers and hand being vibrated on the affected part (Fig. 101).

Shiatsu originally stemmed from osteopathy, a traditional Oriental medical technique which is now quite popular in Japan. However, it has now become an independent art. The basic technique applying to massage is the same as the pressing method used in osteopathy—no new technique has subsequently arisen for such treatment.

In some affected parts, however, a hard pressing method is applied to give an average pressure of 30–50 kilograms per square centimeter with the thumbs. An ambitious research program has recently been carried out into shiatsu and *amma* similar to that into breathing practice in order to assess them in the light of

Fig. 99   **Fig. 100**

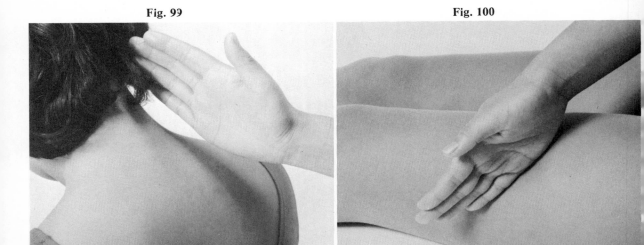

Fig. 101

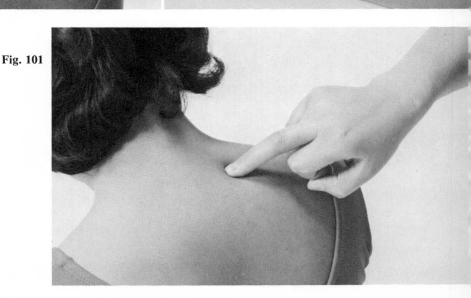

modern Western medical treatment. From the physiological point of view, shiatsu and *amma* were found to have a good effect throughout the body on by enhancing capillary function. It came to light after close study of the effectiveness of these Oriental medical treatments that shiatsu and other related practices greatly improve the circulation of blood and lymph and accelerate metabolism. Therefore, after receiving such Oriental treatment, one feels greatly envigorated.

It is interesting to note that we naturally rub or slap stiff parts of our bodies with the hand, even though we have not been taught to do so. More important facts on the impact of massage treatment were found from other recent clinical research. There is a theory that there must be a close relationship between internal organs and the surface of the body. If stimuli are directed onto the surface of the body, then the resultant impulses are immediately conveyed to deep-lying organs

Fig. 102   Tsubo and Their Manipulation Purposes

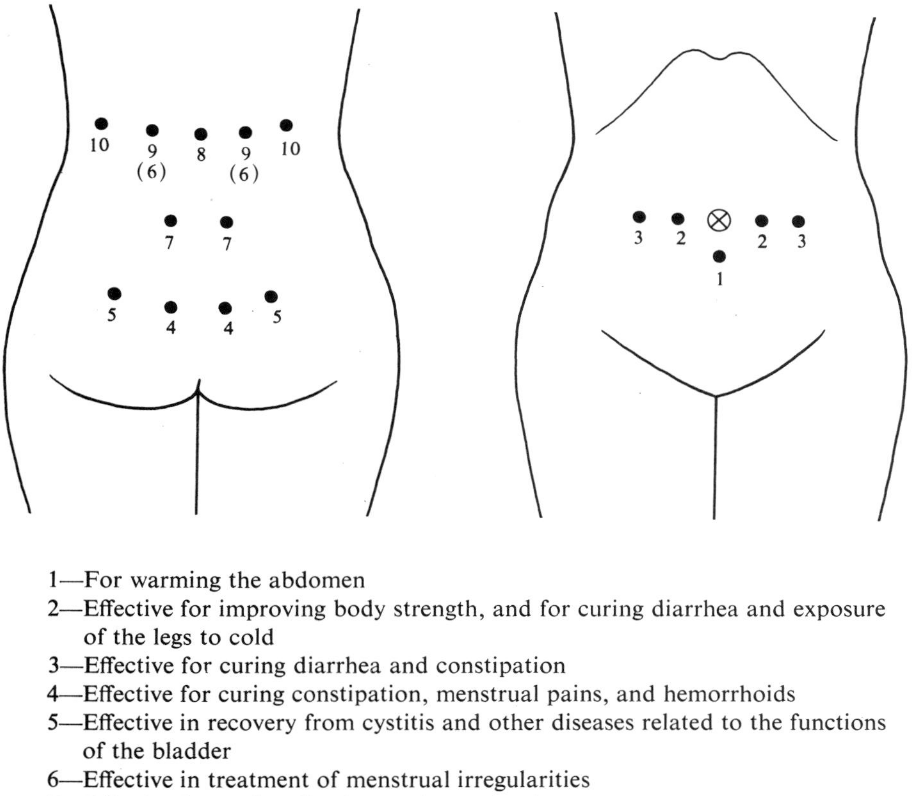

1—For warming the abdomen
2—Effective for improving body strength, and for curing diarrhea and exposure of the legs to cold
3—Effective for curing diarrhea and constipation
4—Effective for curing constipation, menstrual pains, and hemorrhoids
5—Effective in recovery from cystitis and other diseases related to the functions of the bladder
6—Effective in treatment of menstrual irregularities
7—Effective for curing diarrhea and constipation
8—Useful for strengthening body power and improving body condition; also effective for treatment of hip pains
9—Effective for strengthening body power, and curing hip pains
10—Effective for eliminating fatigue and hip pains

and strengthen their functions.

Medical experts in the Orient from about one thousand years ago appreciated this fact and utilized the principle in the treatment of various diseases. However, it is only recently that such ideas have come to the attention of Western medicine. Malfunctions of internal organs usually surface in particular areas called "Head's zones" which are distributed all over the body.

One of these Head's zones is located on the back just behind the stomach, which is called "Mizoochi." Head's zones are in fact identical to the "Tsubo" found in Oriental medicine.

It is certain that shiatsu treatment, like breathing exercises, is very effective for alleviation or recuperation from diseases which are incurable by Western medicine. It would be a mistake, however, to think that diseases incurable by Western medicine could be successfully treated by this application of Oriental medicine. It can hardly be expected that these would be any effect on serious diseases such as cancers, sarcomas, and serious conditions such as phthisis, syphilis, dysentery, cholera, typhoid fever, contagious skin diseases and other epidemic diseases. It is also difficult to completely cure diseases such as thrombosis, embolism, and softening of the brain resulting from brain hemorrhage and hardening of the arteries. But, it is certain that with such diseases as neurotic depression, autonomic imbalance, neuralgia, muscular pains and numbness, remarkable cures can be effected with these treatments. It is said that the treatments are very useful for improvement of health and beauty and for recovery from impotence.

Massage and shiatsu treatment

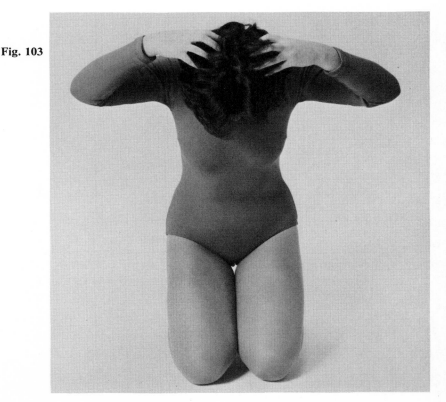

Fig. 103

Head

Insert the fingers of both hands deep into the hair and lightly massage the scalp (Fig. 103). Rub with the inside of the fingers, describing a circle and massage the whole of the surface of the scalp for 50–100 rounds in one session. The treatment stimulates the brain functions and also stimulates the hair roots, preventing baldness and formation of gray hairs.

On completion of massage, brush the hair several times. Also, apply pressure to the back, top and sides of the head with the tips of the fingers. This is an effective treatment for headache, heaviness in the head and occipital neuralgia.

Neck

Knead the musculature of the back of the neck from the top downward with the fingers of both hands placing the palms over the ears (Fig. 104). Repeat this 50–100 times for each round, and on completion, press against both sides of the neck with the fingers; lean your head backward while inhaling and forward while exhaling (Fig. 105). Then again knead the back of the neck ten times. This treatment is effective for treatment of headache, congestion of the brain and ricks in the neck.

When suffering from a rick in the neck, press hard against the musculature diagonally linking throat and ear and massage repeatedly. When pains in the throat are experienced, lightly press the musculature between throat and collar bone. You should find that the pains will abate.

Fig. 104   **Fig. 105**

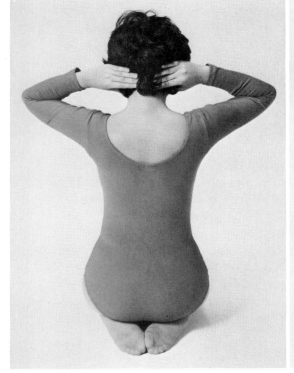
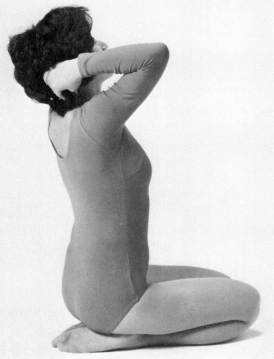

Fig. 106

Fig. 107

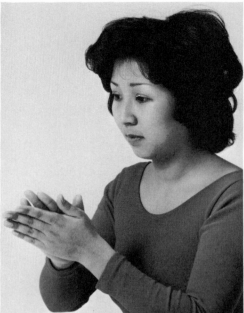

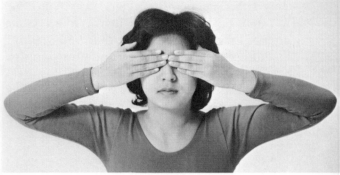

Fig. 108

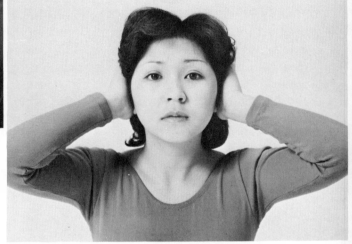

Face

Rub the hands together in order to produce frictional heat (Fig. 106) and then gently rub around the nose, eyes, forehead and ears repeatedly (Fig. 107). Remember to describe circles when patting. Do this thirty-six times for one round. You will find that the parts being rubbed become red and a sense of relief will be felt.

Next, cover your ears with the palms and tap the back of the head using the middle finger covered by the index finger, with the other fingers curled in. This will produce a drumming sound. Repeat this thirty-six times for one round (Fig. 108).

During the final round, press hard against both ear passages with the thumbs for a short time. Repeat this three times. This is very useful for removing wrinkles from your face, and for keeping a healthy complexion. It is also effective for stimulating the functions of the ear and preventing them from losing their function. Lightly press below the ear lobes with the thumbs or index fingers toward the center of the head. This is effective for reducing facial tic.

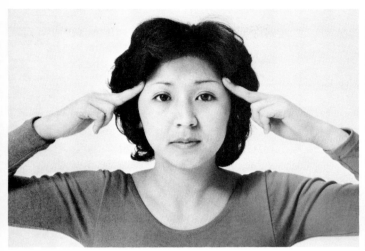

Fig. 109

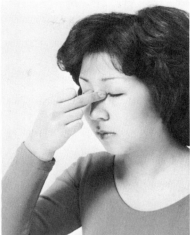

Fig. 110

Eyes

Knead the forehead and hair margin above the ears up and down and to left and right with the eyes in the center (Fig. 109). Repeat this thirty times for one round. Press the temples with the thumbs or index and middle fingers and knead lightly thirty-six times.

Finally place the index finger of one hand between the eyebrows, and the middle finger and thumb of the same hand into the depressions of the each side of the base of the nose adjacent the eyes while closing the eyes, and gently knead (Fig. 110). Repeat this thirty-six times for one round. Having finished, you will find that your eyes will become bright.

This practice is effective for treating headache, dizziness, and various eye diseases. All elementary schools in Shizuoka Prefecture in central Japan adopt this exercise for their pupils who undertake this massage three times every day involving a total of three minutes. It is applied as a means of preventing pseudo-myopia.

Gums

Artificially cause your teeth to chatter for about fifty mouth movements. Hold the forehead with the right hand and the underside of the jaw with the left hand, and continue by changing hands alternately. You will find that a large quantity of saliva will fill your mouth. Rinse the inside of your mouth with this saliva several times, and run your tongue over the back of the teeth which are inundated by the flow of this saliva. Then, swallow the saliva in three stages. It has been shown that the flow of saliva is very effective in treating decayed teeth, pains in the throat and for curing halitosis. It is furthermore believed that artificially causing the teeth to chatter is very effective in stimulating the brain. This also helps a great deal in promoting the development of the brain and is an effective means of preventing senile dementia.

Fig. 111

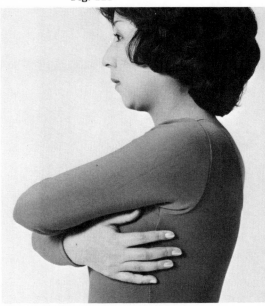

Breast

Place the palm of the right hand on the left side of the breast. Place the tip of the middle finger on the left side of the body some 6 centimeters below the axilla keeping all five fingers slightly separated, and position them between the ribs (Fig. 111). Keep the palm fixed on that breast and rub it lightly fifty times. After this massage, move the hand 5 centimeters downward and rub the side of the breast another fifty times. Knead the entire left breast slightly with the palm hundred times up and down.

Next, change hands and use the left hand to rub the right breast in the same way. This massage is believed to be very effective in recovering from pains of the breasts and in developing beautiful female breasts.

Abdomen

Lightly knead the abdomen from top to bottom with the palm of the right hand and from left to right, with the navel in the center, 50–100 times. Remember not to knead the abdominal region in the reverse direction or keen bellyache may result.

Next, again knead with both palms around the navel (Fig. 112). Remember that both palms should be vibrated while carrying out the massage. After a few minutes, remove both hands from the abdomen and cover the abdomen to avoid undue exposure. This massage is very effective for strengthening the functions of the digestive organs and relieving fatigue in the waist. Press steadily on both sides of the navel (at a position some 3 centimeters on the left and right sides thereof) with both thumbs. This is useful for treatment of chronic gastritis and diarrhea.

Fig. 112

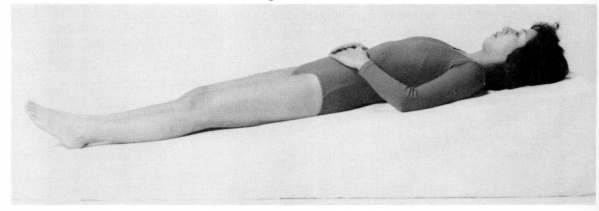

Behind Waist

Place four fingers except the thumb on each side of the coccyx, turn the thumb toward the front of the waist and open four fingers in order to cover as wide a space as possible. Rub the back lightly up and down hundred times for one round. This exercise is effective for treating pains in the waist and kidney disease.

Firmly press each side of the coccyx with the middle fingers. This is beneficial for the treatment of impotence (Fig. 113).

Between Thumb and Index Finger

There is a "Tsubo" called "Gōkoku" (LI-4) in the cavity between thumb and index finger (Fig. 114). Keen pain is felt when pressing this "Tsubo" with the thumb of the other hand. Press this "Tsubo" and relax, repeating hundred times (Fig. 115).

This treatment is very effective for curing toothache, pains in gums and throat, buzzing in the ears and neuralgia of the arms.

Sanri no Tsubo on the Arm

There is a firm "Tsubo" called "Sanri" (LI-10) found on the arm and is located in the musculature of the elbow joint (Fig. 114). Apply pressure to this "Tsubo"

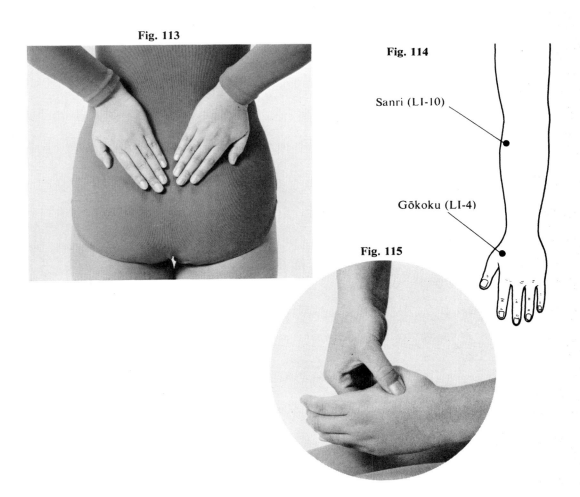

Fig. 113

Fig. 114

Sanri (LI-10)

Gōkoku (LI-4)

Fig. 115

using the hand of the other arm hundred times. This is very effective for treatment of neuralgia of the arms, tonsilitis and rash.

Behind Knees

Apply pressure to the tendon in the musculature behind the knee hundred times for each leg for one round (Fig. 117). This "Tsubo" is called "Ichū" (BL-54) as shown in Fig. 116 and its massage is very effective for treatment of knee pains and sciatic neuralgia, and cramps of the calves.

Knees

Place the palms on the kneecaps and massage the rims of the kneecaps with the fingers hundred times for one round. Lift the palms and knead the knee with the tips of the fingers hundred times (Fig. 118). This treatment is effective for recovering wearyness in the knees and fatigue in the knee joints.

Fig. 116

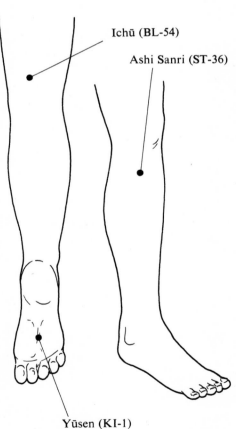

Ichū (BL-54)

Ashi Sanri (ST-36)

Yūsen (KI-1)

Fig. 117

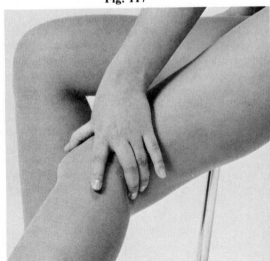

Fig. 118

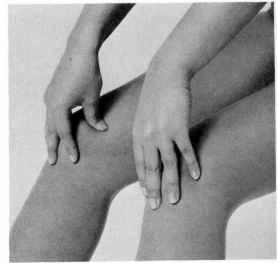

Fig. 119   **Fig. 120**

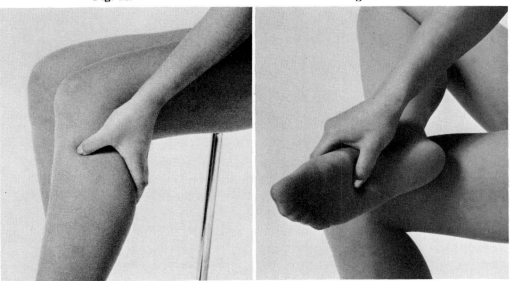

Ashi Sanri

The "Tsubo" called "Ashi Sanri" (ST-36) is located slightly off the tibia some 10 centimeters below the kneecap (Fig. 116). Press this "Tsubo" hard with the thumbs and simultaneously rub on the right and left sides hundred times (Fig. 119). This is a very effective treatment for realizing longevity, eliminating fatigue throughout the body and relieving indigestion. It is highly recommended for treatment of various stomach and intestinal troubles and diabetes as well as neuralgia of the legs.

Sole of the Foot

There is a big "Tsubo" called "Yūsen" (KI-1) in the center of the arch of each foot (Fig. 116). First, press the "Yūsen" of the left foot with the thumb of the right hand hundred times. Then change the hand and foot and press a further hundred times on the "Yūsen" of the right foot with the thumb of the left hand (Fig. 118). This treatment is very effective for treatment of women's disorders, insomnia, heart ailments, and headache.

Mental Attitude for Undertaking Breathing Exercise

Notwithstanding the technological advances made by Western medicine, substantial problems remain be resolved by Oriental medical techniques. There are those who are critical of traditional Oriental treatments, disparaging them as superstitious beliefs or old wives' tales, and some have actively campaigned against the secret therapies. These people, however, really do not know the true meaning of scientific therapy in the Western sense. If in performing these breathing and auxiliary exercises, you maintain a critical attitude with respect to Oriental medicine, then no satisfactory results can be expected regardless of how diligently the exercises themselves are performed.

As was previously mentioned, various studies have been conducted on the effectiveness of Japanese and Chinese breathing therapies, and the results of this research have been published. This type of therapeutic treatment has proved to have remarkable effect, even on those incurable diseases which did not respond to medication, and has improved the health and extended the life of those patients to whom it has been administered. Unlike Western medicine and surgery, these exercises do not cost much.

The undergoing of a program of breathing therapy is both more simple and less expensive than Western style therapeutic treatment. Therefore, if you are suffering from a diseases which Western medicine has been unable to cure, you should try regular breathing exercise with a firm belief and strong determination that you are going to recover from the disease.

Exercise Every Day for First Three Months

It takes a long time to be cured of diseases which are the result of many months and years of intemperate living. It may be difficult to effect remission of diseases which have for years been invading the body and strengthening their hold on the occasion of lowered resistance. Furthermore, since breathing therapy is designed to influence the inside of the human body and affected parts thereof directly, it is not sufficient merely to master the order and methods of the postures and exercises; those who practice the therapy also must master its secrets, such as learning to direct "Ki" throughout the body.

Breathing therapy was originally developed to improve patients' general physical condition and strength by affecting the entire body. Unlike Western therapeutic techniques, it does not seek to achieve the immediate cure of a particularly afflicted part of the body in a limited period of time. The principal objectives of the therapy remain the maintenance of balance within the body and improvement in the condition of major internal organs. This therapy is said to be slow but steady and thorough. Exercisers should, therefore, bear in mind that practice should be carried out prudently, but with firm determination. They should not abandon their goals half way.

It is difficult to say that all problems will be resolved within three months after initiating these exercises on a regular basis. It may safely be said, however, that some substantial progress should be apparent after three months of training have been conducted in accordance with the rigorous programs of breathing therapy introduced in this book. If you recognize the slight changes or improvements in your health which occur while performing these exercises, then your confidence in the program will be strengthened and you will be able to persevere. True health, however, can be attained and maintained only through continued performance of these exercises.

Performance of breathing exercise must be organized

Remember that when you set out to learn something difficult, it is best to start with the easiest aspect and proceed gradually to the more difficult aspects in due course. If you wish to attempt to master the "Unki" method while you are still in the preparatory phase, you will have difficulty. You must realize that the program of exercises is arranged in a sequential order. You must design your own training schedule, giving due consideration to the stage of your own development.

Breathing therapy may be divided roughly into three stages.

1) Preparatory period

This is the period between the point when the exerciser decides to master the therapy and the point at which the exercisers have come about midway in mastering the secrets of regulating their breathing. This period is devoted to the learning of the various patterns of basic breathing exercise. Special effort is required to shift from an ordinary breathing pattern, characterized by quick, heavy, short-interval respiration, to a pattern characterized by slow, flexible respiration.

2) Transition period

This period extends until the difficult "Unki" method (principal method for carrying "Ki" throughout the body) has been mastered. Legend has said that this period is as difficult for beginners as crossing a dangerous river on an unstable suspension bridge. The trick is to get the "Ki" to run throughout the body, but if you make a serious mistake in judgment while learning this lesson, you may lose the opportunity to achieve truly deep comprehension of the breathing therapy. Mastering the technique is likely to take a substantial period of time and considerable practice.

3) Period in which "Unki" is employed positively

Having mastered the technique for directing "Kimyaku" throughout the body, and having become familiar and comfortable with all of the basic breathing exercises, focus your attention on learning the technique for circulating "Ki" and concentrating it in affected parts of the body in order to positively promote the therapeutic effects of the exercise. In so doing, the splendid effectiveness of breathing therapy will be explicitly demonstrated. Wonderful results are assured to all those who perform this exercise.

An Effective Short Cut in Undergoing Breathing Training Is to Set a Target or Goal in Each Stage and to Concentrate on Achieving It

Beginners often become bored after practicing the monotonous exercises for even a rather short time, say three to five minutes, and if they are confronted with even a small problem in the process of performing routine exercises, they give up easily.

Those who have progressed to the study of more advanced techniques tend to discontinue their practice midway through, not because of boredom, but rather because of some consequence of the breathing exercises. Even those people who seem to have a sufficiently strong desire to regain the vitality of youth or to recuperate from chronic diseases and become healthy, often abandon their exercises because they are insufficiently committed to the rigorous exercising training schedule. It is recommended, therefore, that those who desire to master the breathing therapy should resolve that they are going to continue the exercises with the same will and resolve as that required of a martial man facing the enemy hosts.

The best way to persevere is to divide the breathing therapy into several sections in order that those performing the exercises may become familiar with them. This will eliminate any questions about the exercises and their effects, so that those performing the exercises will not experience any sense of frustration and will not waste time attempting to overcome difficulties which might otherwise arise during the course of the exercise. In concrete terms, beginners should establish a weekly or monthly schedule for a daily training program in order to proceed smoothly with the exercises and to concentrate on their control aspects.

Steps to Be Taken in Adjusting to Breathing Therapy

When taking exercise for therapeutic purposes, no particular clothes or tools are required. It is permissible to perform the exercises whenever and wherever the exerciser can find sufficient time and space to do so. The effectiveness of these exercises will increase in proportion to the time expended and the number of repetitions performed. Opportunities for performance of the exercises abound in daily life. For instance, when rising in the morning, before going to bed at night, during a ten-minute recess after lunch, at the railway station, while waiting for a commuter train or even during a short work break in the office while sitting at a desk. There are a particularly large number of opportunities to perform the basic breathing exercises of Types 3, 4 and 5 and Step 1.

Once you have thoroughly mastered the basic principles of breathing therapy, you need not pay particular attention to mastering form and attitude. Even if you assume unusual postures while exercising, you may be able to achieve acceptable results.

Remember that all exercisers should refrain from excessive smoking and drinking while pursuing a course of breathing therapy. They should also avoid participation in gambling games and in general, should avoid leading an intemperate life such as keeping late hours. Unless these injunctions are observed, the effects of the therapy will be dissipated. Therefore, those who desire to have their physiques strengthened and to thereby gain longevity and eternal youth should be moderate in all things. If you master the breathing therapy, there will be no room in your life for vices such as those described. This is because breathing therapy effects fundamental changes in the character of those performing it.

Conclusion

Because the Oriental breathing method described above tends to appear vague and imprecise, it is not particularly appealing to the present generation. Therefore, I have spent about ten years carefully experimenting with the method in order to confirm its effects and better explain how and why it works. I believe that I have succeeded in this and that I have developed a technique more suitable for men in the modern age.

Idea of new method of respiration

A change of mental condition may manifest itself physically through any of a number of symptoms, i.e., paleness or blackness in the face, a change in the appearance of the eyes, distortion of the mouth, or weeping. However, even before these physical symptoms appear, a corresponding change in respiratory and circulatory functions of the body may be observed. It has already been established that the rate of respiration, heart rate, blood pressure, galvanic skin responses (GSR), etc. will fluctuate in accordance with even slight changes in emotional state. Specifically, when you feel well or receive a pleasant stimulus, the number of respirations and the number of heart beats per minute show a decrease.

This coincides with the theory of Carl Gustav Jung (1875–1961) that, unlike unpleasant stimuli which are closely associated with various physical reactions, pleasant stimuli are received passively, without marked response. Muscle tension is closely related to displeasure and muscle relaxation is closely related to pleasure. This applies to involuntary muscles as well. In reaction to pleasant stimulus, involuntary muscle tissue relaxes rather than contracts. This fact contradicts traditional psychological theory, but Dr. Jung proved it in his laboratory.

During the first week after birth, the physiological mechanism of human respiration is characterized by a respiration cycle of approximately forty times per minute and a ventilatory volume of about 498 milliliters per minute and a tidal volume of about 15 milliliters. If subsequent development is healthy, lung function will show an annual increase, reaching a peak in vital capacity at twenty to twenty-three years of age. After hitting the peak, capacity will decrease gradually. The figures show that old men, sixty-six years of age or older, have less capacity than children nine years of age (see p. 23). In females, lung function exhibits a sharp decrease during the mid-forties, about ten years earlier than in males.

I have discussed, therefore, how to prevent aging and achieve a healthier condition. In particular, emphasis must be placed on the lengthening of the period of inspiration and on increasing abdominal pressure. Generally speaking, respiration is conducted by moving the diaphragm and then inhaling or exhaling. And also the diaphragm plays an indispensable role in increasing the pressure inside the abdominal cavity by cooperating with the musculature of the abdominal region. This pressure is found to change in parallel with the changes of posture on the past of exercisers. It also changes as the result of straining while bracing oneself using the abdominal musculature and from applying external pressure to the abdominal region as is done in physical treatment.

The pressure inside the abdominal region can therefore be controlled by the will of exercisers whenever and wherever they wish, with the diaphragm, abdominal muscles and the musculature inside the abdominal wall each making their contribution.

According to clinical researches by Dr. F. A. Gibbs and Dr. E. L. Gibbs, as well as those of Dr. O. Williams of the United States, as the result of a reduction in the blood carbon dioxide partial pressure, the frequency of the appearance of brain waves is found to drastically increase. They explained that carbon dioxide partial pressure also plays a role in reducing the output of brain alpha waves. Dr. E. Gillhorn has also shown that an adequate increase in blood carbon dioxide levels helps to promote reticular formation.

Based on the outcome of these researches, I planned an ambitious experiment to improve the state of mind of the exercisers and also to improve their health. This is attainable by stimulating the limbic system, brain center, and reticular formation in the course of controlling the pressure inside the abdominal cavity.

A trial for new breathing therapy

This trial, aiming at the creation of innovative therapy based on breathing exercise, is endorsed by modern medical scientific theory from the standpoint of time-honored Oriental breathing therapy. This new treatment must be so designed to provide simplicity of application for those seeking uncomplicated therapy and to be employed by medical experts for clinical studies. Three healthy university students, one graduate student, one housewife, and one single woman were selected for testing. These subjects were requested to undergo the following three types of breathing therapy over six months, involving two rounds of breathing exercises every day just prior to going to bed. Each round lasted for about ten minutes, separated by an interval also of ten minutes duration; one complete session therefore involved a total of about thirty minutes.

Breathing Exercise Type 1
Air is quietly inhaled through the nose. After completion of inspiration, puff out a breath through the nose. Breathing is temporarily discontinued for as long as possible while mentally counting the numbers, . . . one, two, three . . . .

The mouth is puckered, followed by expiration over as long a period as possible. (Desirably taking at least three times longer than for inspiration.) It should be remembered while exhaling, to contract the abdominal wall with full strength.

In so doing, all the internal organs within the abdominal cavity are felt to be pushed up toward the thorax. At the same time the anus should be contracted and pulled in.

After exhaling, the abdomen should be smoothly returned to its original position. (In so doing, breathing must be temporarily discontinued.) This is followed by quietly inhaling through the nose. The exercise should be repeated over a ten-minute period.

Breathing Exercise Type 2

Air is quietly inhaled through the nose and the abdomen is contracted. After completing inspiration, numbers are counted mentally, "one, two, three, four, five . . ." while breathing is temporarily discontinued for as long as possible.

While slowly exhaling through the nose, the lower abdomen is expanded, with full strength being thrown into this region.

After fully exhaling, breathing is discontinued while counting mentally up to ten. This exercise is repeated for ten minutes.

Breathing Exercise Type 3

Air is quietly inhaled through the nose, followed by quiet expiration, also through the nose.

While carrying out this breathing exercise, respiration should be continued at a slow pace. While doing so, no movement of chest, abdomen or other parts of the body is allowed except for the up and down movement of the diaphragm (this type of respiration is conducted according to the formula of throwing full strength into the abdominal region), which is analogous to the vertical movement of pistons within an internal combustion engine. This type of respiration is repeated for ten minutes.

These three exercises are designed to be carried out while the exercisers assume a strict posture of sitting squarely on the floor.

Assessment of These Exercises

Assessment was carried out by the following methods.

An electrometabolar was used to check respiratory functions and carbon dioxide metabolism. A transducer was used to check the inner pressure of specially made bellows horses. Measurements were made in a semi-soundproof room at a temperature of 18 degrees centigrade plus or minus 3 degrees.

Experimental Conditions

All subjects of the experiment were required to carry out normal respiration and breathing exercises Types 1, 2 and 3 twice each, and measurements of these tests were taken. Each round of testing lasted some five minutes, with the testing of the breathing exercises Types 1, 2 and 3 being carried out at intervals of ten to fifteen minutes.

There Zen priests of the Sōdō Buddhist Sect acted as a control group, each priest having experienced more than twenty-five years as a bonze monk, each of the control subjects was checked for thirty minutes continuously while assuming the posture of sitting with crossed legs conducive to Zen meditation *(Sanzen)*.

Experimental Results

Regarding the frequency of the respiration cycle, significant differences were found between normal respiration at 15.15 times per minute, breathing exercise Type 1 at 5.5 times per minute, breathing exercise Type 2 at 2.58 times per minute, breathing exercise Type 3 at 1.72 times per minute and Sanzen breathing at 3.23 times per minute.

Regarding minute ventilation volume, although there is no difference between normal respiration and the breathing exercise Type 1 in this respect, significant differences are observed between the breathing exercises Types 2 and 3 and Sanzen breathing.

Almost the same trends are observed between the breathing exercise Type 2 and Sanzen breathing by priests.

With reference to the tidal volume of each breathing exercise, the normal breathing showed quite different results from those of the other exercises.

With regard to RQ, significant gaps are observed between the normal breathing and Type 1, Type 2 and Sanzen breathing exercises, although no large differences are found between the normal and Type 3 breathing.

It has come to light from the experiments that the most ineffective breathing exercise is the normal type, and that the other types, including the Zen priests', are adequately effective.

Dr. Tomio Hirai has explained that the brain alpha waves resulting from the practice of Zen Buddhism are very effective in controlling the autonomic nervous system. The same theories are applicable to the practice of the Types 1, 2 and 3 breathing methods.

It is said that the breathing during Zen meditation involves extension of respiration, breath holding and abdominal pressure, which are believed to be essential features of Oriental breathing methods. It is brought to light that the most efficacious type of breathing technique is that of the Zen Buddhists while they are undergoing Zen meditation.

As mentioned above, the practice of the Sanzen breathing method bears a close relationship to the formation of a healthy state of mind. But it is rather difficult to say that Sanzen breathing method is familiar to contemporary Japanese because of the silent meditation, the posture of sitting with crossed legs and other strict practice methods involved. Therefore, I formulated an entirely new breathing method which can be done in postures of either sitting squarely on a chair or standing upright. This new method is combined with auxiliary exercises which are performed over a short period of time prior to or after the main session.

This breathing method is identical to that which the Buddhists perform during Sanzen breathing from the standpoint of having similar effects in the course

Normal Respiration

Subjects	MRC	MV (l)	TV (l)	MO_2C	MCO_2E	RQ
HA	14.0	11.90	0.85	0.398	0.395	0.9925
TN	15.6	10.50	0.67	0.311	0.307	0.9871
KM	14.3	11.35	0.79	0.307	0.298	0.9706
MN	15.8	9.10	0.58	0.292	0.283	0.9692
KK	16.0	8.05	0.50	0.269	0.256	0.9517
KO	15.2	9.50	0.63	0.286	0.269	0.9406
Mean	15.15	10.07	0.67	0.311	0.301	0.9686

Breathing Exercise Type 1

Subjects	MRC	MV (l)	TV (l)	MO_2C	MCO_2E	RQ
HA	5.9	12.0	2.03	0.354	0.411	1.1610
TN	5.0	9.8	1.96	0.309	0.341	1.1036
KM	5.2	9.0	1.73	0.298	0.327	1.0973
MN	5.9	8.9	1.51	0.272	0.320	1.1765
KK	6.0	8.2	1.37	0.253	0.292	1.1542
KO	5.2	9.0	1.73	0.261	0.295	1.1303
Mean	5.5	9.48	1.72	0.291	0.331	1.1372

Breathing Exercise Type 2

Subjects	MRC	MV (l)	TV (l)	MO_2C	MCO_2E	RQ
HA	2.5	5.2	2.08	0.243	0.252	1.0370
TN	2.5	5.0	2.00	0.271	0.275	1.0147
KM	2.5	5.1	2.04	0.263	0.272	1.0342
MN	2.6	4.7	1.81	0.237	0.245	1.0338
KK	2.8	4.8	1.72	0.252	0.276	1.0953
KO	2.6	4.7	1.88	0.261	0.271	1.0383
Mean	2.58	5.18	1.92	0.254	0.266	1.0422

Breathing Exercise Type 3

Subjects	MRC	MV (l)	TV (l)	MO_2C	MCO_2E	RQ
HA	1.8	3.5	1.94	0.201	0.192	0.9552
TN	1.5	2.9	1.93	0.221	0.203	0.9186
KM	1.6	3.1	1.94	0.209	0.192	0.9187
MN	2.0	3.3	1.65	0.241	0.229	0.9502
KK	1.8	3.1	1.72	0.239	0.223	0.9331
KO	1.6	3.1	1.94	0.243	0.235	0.9671
Mean	1.72	3.17	1.84	0.226	0.212	0.9405

Sanzen Breathing by Zen Priest

Subjects	MRC	MV (l)	TV (l)	MO_2C	MCO_2E	RQ
ZM	3.5	5.2	1.49	0.198	0.250	1.2626
DO	2.8	5.0	1.79	0.179	0.232	1.2961
SM	3.4	5.4	1.59	0.186	0.239	1.2849
Mean	3.23	5.2	1.62	0.188	0.240	1.2812

of passing strength into the lower abdomen, extension of expiration and breath holding, and has similar values for RQ.

Dr. Tomio Hirai has announced his outstanding research work on the relation between respiration and electroencephalographic changes, and Dr. Williams and Dr. Gibbs are currently undertaking clinical studies on this subject. According to these medical experts, in the event of a fall in the venous carbon dioxide partial pressure, the electroencephalographic waves (EEG) shift to a low frequency. If the carbon dioxide partial pressure increases, the EEG waves are found to shift to a high frequency. Thus, their research showed that carbon dioxide partial pressure is a key factor in EEG changes. Carbon dioxide not only has a profound effect upon the respiratory center but also upon a certain stage of reticular formation, and therefore is of great importance in the performance of the respiratory cycle including the hypothalamus. It is still not clear whether any clear relationship between brain waves and changes in blood pressure exist. But, the relationship between functions of the respiratory center and changes in the blood pressure is proved.

It has become clear from this research that EEG activities are accelerated when the respiratory center is excited by external influences such as blood carbon dioxide levels.

From a pharmacological perspective, a stimulant which affects the respiratory system also has the capacity to stimulate brain function. Full investigation and explication of the relationship between the respiratory function and the physiological mechanism of the brain is a subject best left for other medical experts. It is sufficient for our purposes to note merely that breathing therapy influences the brain either through the respiratory center or by direct stimulation of the solar plexus. This further activates the capillary vessels of the vascular system in the abdominal region. This promotes blood circulation, thereby facilitating the rapid absorption of accumulated waste materials and, with the help of major internal organs such as the liver, kidneys and intestines, their elimination from the body. By stimulating the parasympathetic nervous system, breathing therapy also plays a key role in curbing heart rate and in reducing blood pressure. Controlled respiration is a great help in eliminating tension and maintaining tranquility.

In conclusion, if you believe yourself to be suffering from one of following seven symptoms, it is recommended that you immediately perform any of the patterns of breathing exercise in this book.

1. You remain in a somewhat irritated mood, although there is no real reason, or after the initial cause of the irritation has been remedied, or you become offended at the slightest provocation.

2. You continuously feel depressed, although no particular reasons can be identified, or you feel lazy, even though you have made up your mind to do something. You have no hope for the future and all memory of your past is gloomy.

3. You suffer from insomnia, although no particular reasons can be found, or if your sleep is poor and wakeful, so that every morning you wake up

early although there is no particular work to be done.

4. You feel a deep distrust of people around you, although there is no particular basis for such feelings. You feel that all others bear you malice and that you are an outsider.

5. Although you have locked the doors, and turned off the gas and electricity, you still feel uncertain about whether you actually have done so. You often wash clothes that you already have cleaned, and you wash your hands when they are not dirty. You feel irritated unless you clean the room several times a day.

6. Your head always feels heavy, and you suffer from headache. You seem lost in a cloud and are forgetful.

7. You feel clumsy and sense that you are slow in movement and that you fail to react quickly to things moving around you.

All those people to whom even one of these seven symptoms applies may be diagnosed as suffering from a mental disorder. It has been customary to seek psychiatric advice when the above mentioned tendencies continue to appear for over three weeks, but all that the specialist can accomplish is in the way of palliative treatment of symptoms and this does not constitute the resolution of the basic problems. Furthermore, the drugs that you receive undoubtedly will disrupt the function of your digestive organs, but will not cure the underlying disease. Taking the medicines prescribed by these specialists will suppress the symptoms of the disorder, but as soon as you stop taking the medication, you will return to your previous morbid condition. These Western style therapeutic treatments can not permanently and fundamentally cure these mental disorders.

Emotional tension and excitement in modern society are said to cause various nervous diseases and psychosomatic disorders such as peptic ulcer, duodenal ulcer, dermatitis or cutitis, articular rheumatism, respiratory alkalosis, angina pectoris, migraine, hypertension, pollakisuria, dysuria, menstrual disorders, frigidity, impotence, diabetes, Basedow's disease and so on. By examing the following two examples, we can begin to understand how and why these disorders occur.

In the case of hypertension, if repeated psychological and emotional stimuli are received in the cerebral cortex through the primary and secondary signal systems, the nervous system of the cerebral cortex becomes excessively tense. As a result, the inhibitory system in the cerebral cortex does not function and tension builds by positive induction in the contractile tissue of the blood vessels. When this tissue contracts and when the tension persists, the walls of minute blood vessels shrink, and this causes the blood pressure to rise temporarily. Contraction of the arteries of the kidney results in an anemia which will cause the kidneys to create renin, a substance which, when it combines with gamma globulin in the blood, produces hypertensin, raises blood pressure and causes hypertension. The reactionary circle is completed when the rise in blood pressure stimulates the sensory nerve endings in the walls of blood vessels, thereby sending stimuli back to the cerebral cortex.

In the case of peptic ulcer, as in the case of hypertension, abnormal continuous stimulation of the cerebral cortex causes excessive contraction of the muscle fibers within the walls of the stomach and contraction of the blood vessels. As a result, the ability of walls of the stomach to resist the action of digestive fluids within the stomach is reduced. The problem is compounded by the fact that the process of gastric juice secretion is influenced by both reactional and chemical factors. The reactionally induced secretion is a conditioned reflex. The ordinary secretary process is disturbed by irregular diet. This results in an unnecessary secretion of gastric juices. The combination of abnormal secretion and the weakened resistance of the walls of the stomach permit an ulcer to develop quite easily.

Thus, excessive stimulation of the cerebral cortex appears to be among the principal causes of both hypertension and peptic ulcer. The best methods for controlling abnormal stimulation have already been mentioned. The important thing to realize is that it is not impossible to escape from countless stresses continuously placed upon us.

Until now, we have focussed our concentration on external phenomena and external stimuli, and science has made great progress. Now, however, the time has come to focus our undivided attention on the development of our minds. We should exert ourselves to the utmost in an effort to conquer diseases through our own strength.

I honestly hope that you can create a wonderful future by unifying heaven, earth and yourself through the "Ki."

Index

abdominal respiration, 79, 83, 85, 102, 108, 109
acidosis, 20, 29
acupuncture, 30, 100, 135
amma, 100, 138, 139
anemia, 35
angina pectoris, 157
Annetsu method, 135 136
anxiety neuroses, 15
apical breathing, 102
Appaku method, 135 136
arteriosclerosis, 29, 39, 108
arthritis, 117, 118, 122
articular rheumatism, 157
Ashi Sanri, 109, 147
asthma, 122, 124
autonomic imbalance, 140

Basedow's disease, 157
brain hemorrhage, 140
breath counting system, 61
bronchial asthma, 108
bronchial respiration, 19
Buddha, 111
Buddhism, 71, 111
buzzing in the ears, 145

cancer, 104
cardiocentesis, 39
cerebral apoplexy, 61
cholecystitis, 54
cholera, 140
clot, 29
compulsive neuroses, 15
conception vessel, 104, 106
Confuciasm, 71
congestion of the brain, 141
constipation, 28, 54, 113, 141
contagious skin disease, 140
cramp of the calves, 146
cutitis, 157
CV-1, 106, 109
CV-4, 62
cyanosis, 20

cystitis, 141

dermatitis, 157
diabetes, 147, 157
difficulty in breathing, 18
diarrhea, 141, 144
dizziness, 143
duodenal ulcer, 28, 54, 108, 157
dysentery, 140
dyspnoea, 108
dysuria, 157

Ein, 62, 109
embolism, 140
endorphin, 12
enteritis, 28, 108
enteroparesis, 109

facial tic, 142
fetal breathing, 67, 69
Form of Holding a Tiger Down, 45
Form of Three Circles, 40
Form of Three Matches, 43
frigidity, 157
Fu, 66
Fuga, 52, 54
Fukanzazengi, 48
Fukkihō, 68
Fukko no Katachi, 45
Fusoku, 107
Fuzai, 47, 52

gallstone, 109
gastric catarrh, 28
gastric ptosis, 28, 54, 108
gastritis, 28, 144
gastrospasm, 18
Gibbs, E. L., 152, 156
Gibbs, F. A., 152, 156
Gillhorn, E., 152
Gōkoku, 109, 145

Golz's Experiment, 64
governing vessel, 104, 106
GV-20, 106, 109
Gyōga, 52

halitosis, 143
Hanka Fuza, 47, 49
headache, 29, 34, 99, 121, 122, 141, 143, 147, 157
Head's zone, 140
heart disease, 31, 44, 53, 89, 90, 98, 99, 108, 115, 116, 119, 122, 124, 147
heaviness in the head, 141
hemorrhoid, 91, 98, 141
hernia in the intervertebral disc, 117, 118
Hinduism, 71
hip pain, 141
Hirai, Tomio, 154, 155
Hiraza, 51
Hizakuzushizuwari, 51
Hyakue, 106, 109
hypertension, 31, 39, 61, 89, 90, 98, 99, 108, 115, 116, 119, 122, 124, 157, 158
hyperventilation, 16, 17, 19, 34
    alkalosis, 18
    tetany, 17
hypochondriasis, 15
hypotension, 35
hysteria, 15

I, 36, 37, 46
Ichū, 109, 146
impotence, 140, 145, 157
indigestion, 147
insomnia, 108, 147, 156
intestinal catarrh, 28

joint pain, 122
Jūnetsu method, 135
Jung, Carl Gustav, 151

Junki, 102

Kangen, 62
Keisatsu method, 135
Kekka Fuza, 13, 48, 49
Ki, 30
KI-1, 106, 109, 147
kidney disease, 145
Kimyaku, 149
Kisoku, 36, 42, 47, 49, 106, 107
Kizai, 47, 52
knee pain, 146
Kōda method, 135, 137

lame hip, 120, 122
Lao Tze, 12
LI-10, 145
liver trouble, 109
lumbago, 121, 122

Maumann, E., 12
menstrual irregularity, 108, 109, 141, 157
menstrual pain, 141
Mentz, P., 12
migraine, 157
Mizoochi, 140
moxibustion, 30, 100, 135
Musoku, 111

Naikan, 111
Nai San Go, 35, 63
Needham, Walter, 19
Nehan, 111
naphrolithiasis, 54
nervous prostration, 108
neuralgia, 140
    of the arms, 145, 146
    of the legs, 147
neurasthenia, 61
neurotic depression, 140
Nihon Shoki, 12, 65

occipital neuralgia, 141
Ohga, 52
Ohmyaku, 63

Okimyaku, 62

pain in the foot, 29
    in the gum, 145
    in the throat, 141, 143, 145
    in the waist, 145
    of the breast, 144
peptic ulcer, 28, 54, 157, 158
phobia, 15
phthisis, 108, 140
pollakisuria, 157
Prana, 12
proctoptosis, 54
pseudomyopia, 143
pulmonary apiatis, 102
pulmonary respiration, 19
pulmonary tuberculosis, 122
pyelitis, 54

rash, 146
reaction melancholia, 15
Rehwodt, F., 12
renal calculosis, 109
Renmo, 104, 106
rephritis, 36
respiratory alkalosis, 157
rick in the neck, 141

Samādhi, 35
Sanen no Katachi, 40
Sanmai, 62
Sangō no Katachi, 43
Sanri, 145
Sanzen, 154
sarcomas, 140
Satori, 111
schizophrenia, 15
sciatic neuralgia, 146
Seiki, 67, 70
Seiza, 48–51, 64
senile dementia, 143
Sen Ki Nai Kō, 36
shiatsu, 100, 105, 138–140
Shiki, 70
Shinsen method, 135, 138
Shinsoku, 107, 109, 111
Shintoism, 71
Shizen Anza, 48, 49

shortness of breath, 19, 99
softening of the brain, 140
Sokusō, 111
Sokuten principle, 65
ST-36, 109, 147
stiffness in the shoulders, 103
stomachache, 28, 38, 103
Sūsokukan, 62
sutra, 61
syphilis, 140

Taisoku, 67
Tanden, 42
Taoism, 71
Tatehizazuwari, 51
thoracic respiration, 17, 72, 82, 83, 102
thrombosis, 140
Tomo, 104, 106
tonsilitis, 146
toothache, 29, 145
Tsubo, 62
typhoid fever, 140

valsalva, 39
valsalva breath holding, 19, 61, 75, 116

Unki, 149

Williams, 156
Wundt, Wilhelm, 12

Yinki, 65, 66
Yōjōkun, 49
Yōki, 65, 66, 102, 105
Yūsen, 109, 147

Zazen contemplation, 42
Zen, 34, 42, 48, 61, 62, 154
Zengo, 49
Zesoku, 107
Zō, 66, 70
Zoneff, P., 12
Zuisoku, 110, 111